# KRIYA Y_ _

## FOR SELF-DISCOVERY

"This book is deliciously detailed, deep, and elegantly expressed. I cannot recommend it enough to anyone interested in learning Kriya yoga as a more-needed-than-ever method for systematically expanding consciousness."

EVE BAUMOHL NEUHUAS, AUTHOR OF
*THE CRAZY WISDOM OF GANESH BABA*

"Valuable step-by-step instructions for posture, breath, inner gaze, and awareness of subtle perception. Throughout this book, the author's tone rings with encouragement: be curious, trust yourself, all will be revealed."

YOGACHARYA ELLEN GRACE O'BRIAN,
AUTHOR OF *THE JEWEL OF ABUNDANCE*

"In this remarkable book, Dr. Lowenstein shares with great clarity both the profoundly practical knowledge of Kriya yoga and insights he brings to this ancient wisdom through the lens of cutting-edge health science. This book is a real treasure—enjoy!"

JIM CARSON, PH.D., AND KIMBERLY CARSON, MPH, C-IAYT,
COAUTHORS OF *RELAX INTO YOGA FOR CHRONIC PAIN*

"Dr. Lowenstein's Kriya yoga is a gift. It represents the passage of an ancient lineage through his personal apprenticeship with Ganesh Baba into a modern science-based exegesis. In this book, he offers practitioners, from novice to advanced, unique access to an invaluable body of wisdom and practical skills."

CHRIS STAUFFER, M.D., ASSISTANT PROFESSOR OF PSYCHIATRY
AT THE OREGON HEALTH AND SCIENCE UNIVERSITY (OHSU)

"With topics ranging from a neuroscience-based discussion of Dr. Stephen Porges's Polyvagal Theory to an exploration of the impact of Kriya yoga on spiritual development, this book is a must-read for anyone in improving their physical, mental, or spiritual health."

DONNA KIRCHOFF, M.D., FAAP, INTEGRATIVE PEDIATRICIAN

"This book is a beacon for those of us who have goals of solace, gratitude, and peace. Its reading is a smooth, fluid presentation of the discipline of Kriya yoga, and its lessons are stunningly beneficial to the reader."

DONALD E. GIRARD, M.D., PROFESSOR OF MEDICINE EMERITUS
AT THE OREGON HEALTH AND SCIENCE UNIVERSITY
SCHOOL OF MEDICINE

"George Harrison described the sixties and seventies as a 'mini-Renaissance,' and along with its famous geniuses were a number of inspired visionaries working in relative obscurity to combine the best of Eastern wisdom with the perspective of Western science to further the evolution of the human species. And they are ready to share their stories to those seeking more meaningful lives. Keith Lowenstein is one of them."

SCOTT TEITSWORTH, AUTHOR OF
*KRISHNA IN THE SKY WITH DIAMONDS*

"At the same time an introduction to the beautiful science of Kriya yoga for an uninitiated public and a comprehensive manual for experienced practitioners, this book comes at a perfect time in our era when spiritualization is becoming a vital necessity."

CHRISTIAN PILASTRE, KRIYACHARYA (MASTER TEACHER)
AT TRIPOURA YOGA CENTRE

"A disciplined practice, involving breathing exercises, meditation, and posture. In chapters on Kriya yoga's lineage, practice, and scientific and spiritual effects, the authors masterfully explain it, presupposing no previous knowledge of yoga or philosophy."

J. M. FRITZMAN, PH.D., ASSOCIATE PROFESSOR IN THE
DEPARTMENT OF PHILOSOPHY AT LEWIS & CLARK COLLEGE

"Dr. Lowenstein's book has many hints and instructions that can be followed with benefit. He has been a practitioner for forty years and shares his journey in a way that may help us further open ours. It is at once practical and touches deep psychospiritual wells. Something to practice and grow with."

MICHAEL EIGEN, PH.D., PSYCHOLOGIST AND AUTHOR OF
*THE CHALLENGE OF BEING HUMAN*

"This illustrated work offers a grounded and comprehensive view of Kriya yoga's history, theory, and practice, giving new expression to an ancient truth: the power of human breath and posture to affect body, mind, spirit, and heart. A very helpful and easily readable book."

ROBIN BAGAI, PSY.D., LICENSED PSYCHOLOGIST

"Presents easy-to-understand steps to develop a Kriya practice. Although one needs patience in the gradual development of the practice, Dr. Lowenstein mentions how some results can be immediate, and I agree. This is a must-have book for every human. And remember, 'breath control is mind control.'"

MARY K. MCCARTHY, M.D., PAST PRESIDENT
OF THE OREGON PSYCHIATRIC ASSOCIATION

# KRIYA YOGA
## FOR SELF-DISCOVERY

Practices for
Deep States of Meditation

Keith G. Lowenstein, M.D.,
with **Andrea J. Lett, M.A.**

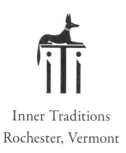

Inner Traditions
Rochester, Vermont

Inner Traditions
One Park Street
Rochester, Vermont 05767
www.InnerTraditions.com

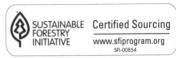

SUSTAINABLE Certified Sourcing
FORESTRY
INITIATIVE www.sfiprogram.org
SFI-00854

Text stock is SFI certified

*This publication contains the opinions and ideas of the author. It is intended to provide helpful and informative material on the subjects addressed in the publication. It is provided with the understanding that the author and publisher are not engaged in rendering medical, health, psychological, or any other kind of personal professional services in the book. If the reader requires personal medical, health, or other assistance or advice, a competent professional should be consulted. The author and publisher specifically disclaim all responsibility for any liability, loss, or risk, personal or otherwise, that is incurred as a consequence, directly, or indirectly, of the use and application of any of the contents of this publication.*

Cataloging-in-Publication Data for this title is available from the Library of Congress

ISBN 978-1-64411-218-2 (print)
ISBN 978-1-64411-219-9 (ebook)

Printed and bound in the United States by Lake Book Manufacturing, Inc. The text stock is SFI certified. The Sustainable Forestry Initiative® program promotes sustainable forest management.

10 9 8 7 6 5 4 3 2 1

Artwork by Lubosh Cech, luboshcech.com (unless otherwise noted)
Text design and layout by Priscilla Baker
This book was typeset in Garamond Premier Pro with Gryffith, Optima, and Futura used as display typefaces

To send correspondence to the author of this book, mail a first-class letter to the author c/o Inner Traditions • Bear & Company, One Park Street, Rochester, VT 05767, and we will forward the communication, or contact the author directly at **kriyabreath.com.**

# Contents

# Foreword

## Andrea J. Lett

Writing a book about yoga is an act of courage and an act of faith. To write about a tradition whose roots are unimaginably resilient, one must possess a fair amount of confidence. It is a bold move for a westerner to offer information about such an ancient practice, and it requires a deep commitment to help it to continue to flourish. Yoga is a multifaceted tradition that contributes sincerely to the spiritual expansion of many peoples and cultures. As a medical anthropologist, I am curious about how particular cultures cultivate spirituality, and as a yoga practitioner, I am continually awed by the potential of yoga to change so many lives.

Yoga's wisdom is somewhat elusive but not because it is secretive; rather, it invites the seeker to embody the appropriate level of awareness wherever they are in their learning. A beginner can achieve results with basic breathing techniques or asanas (postures) just as a seasoned yogi will achieve greater awareness. Within each layer of expansion, the practitioner is allowed to remain where they are while also given enough guidance to move forward.

When I was in middle school, my grandmother taught me Transcendental Meditation, a practice that she and my grandfather practiced daily. It wasn't until college that I came to know yoga and at that time it was considered solely an asana-based practice and was relegated to the realm of physical fitness. Since then, I have studied health, fitness, meditation, medicine, shamanism, and nutrition and found them all to be useful modalities in their own right. However, I found each one to be limited in what it could offer on a path toward wellness and healing. I came to understand that at some point we must become masters of our own universe and turn inward for the answers we seek. I discovered that using a Kriya yoga practice as the way to do that is both simple and complex.

My first lesson in Kriya was to sit up straight, which caused a great deal of discomfort. In working with Dr. Lowenstein over a short time, I began to value the structural shift in my body. As he demonstrated more about the deep connection he had with his own teachers and how Kriya moved through his life, I began to see the differences in the way I felt when I practiced. The more I worked with posture the more comfortable I became in my own body. Many chronic aches and pains from previous injuries began to correct themselves through proper postural alignment. When I incorporated breathing practices, my life shifted exponentially. Breathwork is a subtle art as it is something we rely on automatically. We can easily take it for granted, but when it is focused, it becomes a primary tool for refining our awareness and guiding our innate intelligence in ways that lead naturally to growth, mindfulness, and health. It is not an exaggeration to say that Kriya has altered the course of my wellness in transformational ways.

The material presented here is unlike any other I have come across in my studies of yoga. Initially, while practicing yoga in mainstream Western classes, Kriya was a form I was only aware of in passing. Over the course of a year of study with Dr. Lowenstein, Kriya yoga has become a thread of nourishment feeding the deepest parts of my Self. Kriya is a beautiful and living science that draws wisdom from ancient philosophies and integrates it with contemporary struggles. It is both enduring and evolving. It is a daily invitation to develop a relationship with humanity, to walk in humility and embrace the wonder. The entire Kriya lineage is present when one steps onto this path and teachers do show up when they are most needed.

I truly hope that readers will find this guide to be a useful tool; a lamp to illuminate the path on their journey toward wholeness. It has been a great honor to have been a part of bringing this book to fruition, as studying Kriya has offered me so much. It has shown me time and again that all we call reality lives within us—that we possess the potential to change our lives, to know ourselves, and to be one with all that is.

ANDREA J. LETT holds a BS in neuroscience/nutrition and an MA in medical anthropology/somatic psychology. She is a body-mind wellness practitioner with twenty years of experience practicing and teaching yoga and meditation to kids and adults, postpartum nutrition coaching, somatic therapy, and Zen shiatsu to help people navigate the complexities of post-traumatic stress disorder, or PTSD. She began studying Kriya while working on this book and remains steadfast in her commitment to the practice. Her website is dreajlett.com.

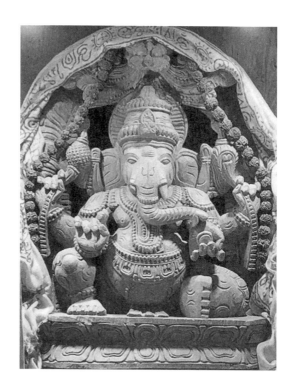

Ganesh is associated with the creative root of the earth, Mother Nature as we experience her. He is also known as the remover of all obstacles. (Photo by Keith Lowenstein.)

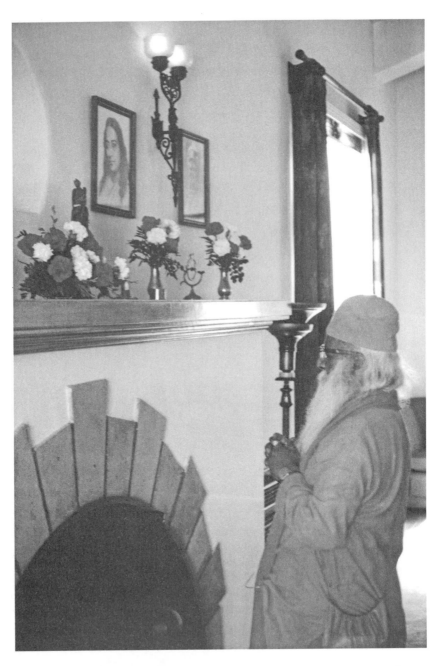

Ganesh Baba inside Yogananda's house in Encinitas, circa 1983. Over the mantle hang pictures of Paramahamsa Yogananda, Sri Yukteswar, and Lahiri Mahasaya among others. The pictures of Paramahamsa Yogananda and Sri Yukteswar are visible in this photograph. (Photo by Keith G. Lowenstein.)

# Acknowledgments

It would take me another volume to begin to scratch the surface of the deep gratitude I have for the many people who have shared a path with me over the years.

Of course, this book would not be possible without the loving generosity of Ganesh Baba's patience, intelligence, fortitude, resilience, strength, humor, tenacity, and fearlessness as he provided a loving stable structure for me to sit still in and breathe. The Kriya line continues to provide inspiration that is woven into this book in a multitude of ways. Over the years I have been influenced by others in the Kriya line, including, Paramahamsa Hariharananda, who provided additional Kriya yoga instruction for me in the early 1980s. Others in the Kriya line with whom my path has crossed and have been influential have included Paramahamsa Prajnananananda, Hilda Charlton, Roy Eugene Davis, and most recently Sri Mukherjee.

It was the love of Roxanne and Jayant Gupta, who brought Ganesh Baba to this country in the late 1970s for a corneal transplant as he was about to lose sight in his only functioning eye. The second attempt at the surgery was successful, and I met him shortly thereafter.

Jayant, Roxanne, Eve Neuhaus, and many others in the Finger Lakes region of New York State provided support for me when I arrived on the scene with Ganesh Baba clearly explaining to me that I would be with him for five years to learn the things that he had to teach me.

This statement proved accurate almost to the day. On the second day of knowing Ganesh Baba he instructed Dan Kraak to give me my first Kriya yoga lesson in posture, which I remember to this day. The first twelve to eighteen months I spent with Ganesh Baba was also spent with Dan, his cats, and my dog, Sheba, who became Ganesh Baba's good friend. During this time, I was afforded much generosity by many around, including Eve, who for a period of time allowed me to treat her home as my own and continues to be a deep and close friend.

A few years later, after completing my medical internship, Jayant provided a haven for my wife (who had also just finished her internship) and me for a week of rest and rejuvenation. The loving support and wonderful food that Jayant provided to us over that week was deeply nourishing to the soul, and the memory of that week continues to warm my heart.

There were many others in the Ithaca area that contributed to the general community around Ganesh Baba, including Kip, Bob and Carol, Kapil, Brenden, Lisa, David and Madeline, Bobby, and Diane, among others. Ganesh Baba and I also spent a few years in New York City where he introduced me to many American friends that he knew from India twenty years earlier. These included Ira Cohen, Ira Landgarten, Karl Hartig, and Hallie Goodman to name a few. In addition, we taught Kriya yoga class typically once a week just off the Bowery on Spring Street in what is now SoHo. Although some of these individuals have passed on to the other side, I expect many who are still in their body are still practicing Kriya. Those attending regularly in New York City include Johnathan, Fred, Perry, Robert, Lois, Barbara, Michael, Len, Gale, Andrea, Mama Dog, Randy, Carol, Jenny, Michela, Alex John, Dr. G, and many more. There are quite a few individuals who live in California, including Amy Steiner and Dulal as well. There was also written correspondence with many others whom Ganesh Baba loved and stayed in touch with around the world, and he also has students in France, including Christian and Corinne, that continue to teach Kriya yoga. This book is an invitation to any past students of Ganesh Baba to get back in contact.

Of course, no book would be complete without giving gratitude to the teachers of the world. Those who love humanity, nature, and knowledge and are driven to share from the heart. As a young man I met an old friend of my grandfather's on the street corner one day. While waiting to cross the street he looked me in the eyes with great intent and said, "Know what you talk. Don't talk what you know." The meaning being to share the knowledge that you have embodied in one way or another. Do not just recite facts to fill the airwaves or your ego. It is my hope that this book will meet those expectations. My path has been blessed by having many teachers from the time I was a small boy. No matter where my path brought me there was a teacher, mentor, friend, family member, or aspect of Mother Nature to help along the way. I would like to acknowledge my deep gratitude to all those individuals who shared some of their time and attention with me.

During the two years that it took to discuss the book, outline it, write it, illustrate it, and get it to the publisher I had the interest and support from many including Bella, Sita, Eve, Roxanne, Jayant, Corinne, Christian, Jim, Nancy, and Duncan as well as a number of interested beginning practitioners all of whom I am privileged to know. Lyndsey Anderson who has been studying Kriya since 2017, provided some assistance with the final edit of the manuscript. The manuscript also benefited greatly from early editing suggestions by Nancy Yeilding, an editor who materialized at the precise moment she was needed. The final editing credit goes to Meghan MacLean, who brought the project to completion with extraordinary clarity and grace. Lubosh Cech provided the illustrations to help illuminate the details, and Michelle Cruzel shares her wonderful photographs of Ganesh Baba from a time he was in France. All contributed their wisdom and compassion in many ways that added depth to the publication.

While I was pursuing my education and practicing as a physician in Oregon, my cowriter and now good friend, Drea Lett, was busy learning neuroscience, hatha yoga, and perfecting her writing technique. I had been looking for a cowriter for approximately six years, and Drea arrived on the scene to ensure that I would follow Ganesh Baba's request to write about "Human Holistics," which really is the art and science of Kriya yoga.

The writing of this book has been a process and without Drea the book would likely still be residing in my mind. In fact, Drea's arrival, brought about through a series of synchronistic events, put in place the next generational transfer of Kriya via manuscript writing. Ganesh Baba used this technique to teach many of his students, including Eve and me. Ganesh Baba himself wrote volumes at the behest of his last Kriya teacher Sri Tripura.

Drea's commitment to this project was firm from the start. She had no qualms directing me to write more about this or that subject to help further illuminate aspects she found to be overly complex or too vague. Drea's creativity helped illuminate this manuscript in a myriad of ways as she embraced the teachings and began to experience the techniques' transformational abilities. I am humbled by her fortitude, curiosity, and compassion as she now moves forward teaching others the joys of breath and posture of this Kriya line. She has been instrumental in bringing these teachings to the printed page, and anyone one who finds grace within these pages should know how it came to be.

Ehud Sperling, president of Inner Traditions, initially asked me to write a book almost forty years ago. At the time he asked for "a small book on meditation." I was twenty-two at the time and did not feel I had the knowledge or experience to write such a book. Despite his encouragement I politely declined, and he began the process of working with Ganesh Baba and Eve on a book that was a challenge to finish with Ganesh Baba around as the editing process often followed Ganesh Baba's insistence that they start all over again. Eve did eventually write a book about the years with Ganesh Baba and it came out approximately thirty years later.

Ganesh Baba was very clear in his instruction to me. He said, "I am giving you Human Holistics. You must now go to medical school and put it forth." We had been working together for little more than a year

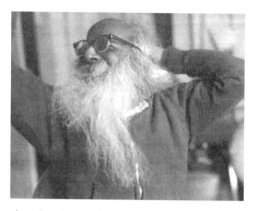

Ganesh Baba, North Albany Street, Ithaca, NY, 1981.
(Photo by Keith G. Lowenstein.)

at that point in time, and I had already been taking classes in anatomy and physiology at the local community college to help me better teach Kriya. During that year we were spending most of our time together in half of a small carriage house outside of Ithaca on a farm. It was a fairly quiet and isolated place to be. Perfect for two young men, cats, a dog, and an eighty-five-plus-year-old Kriya yogi to spend time together learning Kriya, drinking chai, making dahl and rice, sitting up straight, breathing, and not infrequently watching the sunrise after a night of Kriya.

Speaking of chai and dahl, my absence has been clearly evident in our kitchen, the hearth of our home. I have deep love, gratitude, and respect for my family and their help over the decades. During the process of writing this book my wife, Shelley, and my two daughters stepped forward to provide extra assistance to the household as my attention became subsumed in the chapter of the moment. Once the manuscript was ready to go to the publisher, it was back to the kitchen as we planned to cook a dinner for some new friends, Jim and Kimberly, who came our way via the Kriya path. It is only the generosity of all these individuals that allowed these words to come forth in this book.

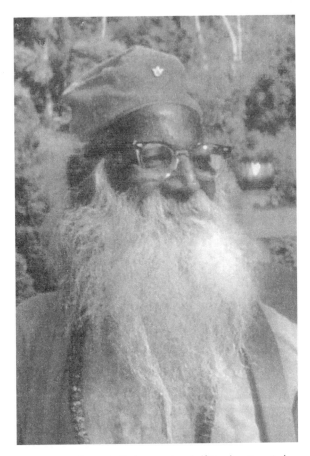

Figure I.1. Ganesh Baba at the Self-Realization Lake Shrine, early 1980s. (Photo by Keith G. Lowenstein.)

## INTRODUCTION
# Welcome to the Kriya Path

The passage of time seems to possess an uncanny way of marinating knowledge and transforming it into seeds of wisdom. It was some forty years ago, in the springtime, that I first met Ganesh Baba.

Ganesh Baba was a lively, spirited Indian man in orange sadhu clothes and a genius in his own right. His genius was that he had a keen ability to look at a variety of yogic and meditation techniques, philosophies, and experiences and distill them down to their most essential parts. He then combined them in the ways that made them simpler to use. This also made them surprisingly effective and helped with the dissemination of this knowledge in English, currently the most accessible language of Western science.

His first task was finding English words to take the place of what historically had been expressed in Sanskrit, Bengali, Hindu, or other languages of the Indian subcontinent because many of these terms have a variety of definitions when translated into English and often lead to misunderstandings by westerners. In general, he succeeded, although in this most recent reiteration of Kriya yoga, the terms have been adjusted based on cultural changes and understandings. These adjustments are consistent with how Ganesh Baba taught his students.

Once he removed obtuse Sanskrit terms that could easily swallow a student's attention and distract from the ease of the practice, he simplified complicated routines of multiple postures, various perceived

1

austerities, long hours in isolation, rituals, faiths, and superstitions, presenting them in a clear and systematic fashion. He hoped to inspire the younger generations as well as reach the elders and insisted this knowledge be spoken about and written in English to reach the largest possible audience. His intention was to bring what was then the esoteric practice of yogic meditation to lay people of the Western world. There were many taboos surrounding who could be taught these techniques, which had previously been largely relegated to monks. However, Ganesh Baba started offering these practices to householders and individuals. And, more generally, these restrictions have been slowly fraying and breaking down over the past 150 years.

Ganesh Baba was educated in British India. He was a householder himself working in business and always studying science. He lived through India's independence and became a monk at around forty years of age. He had many teachers and gleaned from each of their teachings a highly synthesized model that integrated the science of his generation with the ancient philosophies of the Vedanta (a school of Indian philosophy). What makes his contribution unique was that he distilled the practice so as to preserve its essence while enhancing its efficacy. Ganesh Baba was fully aware of the challenges of the westerner's plight: that our attention span suffers from many distractions. He was also acutely aware of the changes in society and envisioned Kriya as a way to help spiritualize the population and help spark a revolution! He saw the hippy movement as the second coming, a new consciousness that opened the world to a larger awareness, but he also saw the increase in drug use as a potential distraction.*

Ganesh Baba's wish was to see a shift in the collective consciousness of humanity. He hoped that Kriya would be a light for others to follow toward inner peace and awakening. Modalities like Kriya yoga provide self-regulatory methods needed by all throughout the world. These basic skills can offer both adults and children a foundation for

*See appendix 1 for more information on the history and use of psychedelics in meditation.

holistic living and help them develop their innate abilities, self-love, and creative expression. These practices provide a basis for well-being as well as healthy coping mechanisms for stress reduction.

Within a few days of our meeting, Ganesh Baba proclaimed I would soon be teaching others. A thought I quickly put out of my mind, but by that autumn I was teaching classes next to him. Before the end of our first year together he was instructing me to transfer the teachings to visiting students who were coming for instruction from other countries. It was from that point forward that he placed me in the primary teaching role for some students. I've not taken the responsibility lightly and have provided mostly private instruction over the years. I spent about five years with Ganesh Baba and was his last main student. It is now time to begin the transfer of these teachings to the next generation and to follow the instructions of Ganesh Baba's teachers to leave "footprints on the sands of time," as Longfellow once put it. It is only through our relationship with others that we can all hopefully move forward on the evolutionary path that the master yoga practitioners see as Self-Realization, or the direct experience of the essence of all religion. This book is my humble attempt to honor the teachers in the various lineages that have contributed to my own Kriya journey.

In recent years, I have come across many volumes written about Kriya yoga, many of them reproduced to reflect as carefully as possible the works of earlier Kriya yoga teachers. As a practitioner, I am interested in this material but have found it to be dense and complex beyond what is necessary for beginners on this path, which may be a large part of why this practice and others like it are regarded as secret. Part of the motivation for writing this book is to make Kriya more accessible and user-friendly so that anyone interested in Self-Realization via Kriya may achieve it. All the Kriya yoga techniques discussed in this book were taught openly by Ganesh Baba. This is not the case in all the Kriya lines. In writing this book the wishes of each branch of the Lahiri line were respected with regards to not publishing material that is unique to their line and that they only share with those who have been initiated within their group.

Kriya yoga is a technique that can help humans accelerate their spiritual evolution. Of course, we must practice regularly with focus, intensity, and a deep inner yearning in order to experience our infinitely dimensional universe. One element that Ganesh Baba and I spent a considerable amount of time exploring was that of spiritualization: what it is and how to achieve it. Spiritualization is the activation of our acutely specialized and highly evolved central nervous system, which acts as an antenna for refining energies that exist beyond the physical body. It is thought to be more like a lightning rod for *metaphysical* awareness. We will continue to explore this concept through the art and science of Kriya yoga, as it is essential for the evolving consciousness of humanity.

At this point in our human history we have a unique opportunity to change our future and that of future generations. With the internet making information instantaneously available to the masses, we can share knowledge like never before. We also have a rare responsibility to do more with what we have in a way that impacts the planet and the people on it in positive, life-affirming ways. Kriya yoga is one such way. It is a practice of fine-tuning and "magnetizing" the central nervous system toward synchronization with subtle energies and vibrations that are unseen with the physical eye but perceived nonetheless. What we have now, thanks to Ganesh Baba's work, is an accelerated physiological technology of Kriya yoga.

Although yogic meditation predates Buddhist practice, it has not gained the same attention in the West. Similarities between the two paths are present and build upon one another. All Indo-Buddhist traditions are similar in practice and theory but differ in practical emphasis and philosophical descriptions. It was Buddha who first outlined the concept of the "middle way." Buddha's approach to meditation has a slightly more cognitive focus in the West and has garnered a social and community-oriented tradition. In this way, it has given foundation to the practice of mindful awareness, or mindfulness.

Mindfulness is an act of integrating aspects of the body and mind, or body-mind; however, achieving it is often left somewhat to the serendipitous nature of the individual and their environment. The length of time needed to achieve tangible spiritual results with a mindfulness practice can often take quite a bit longer than focused yogic meditation practice.

Mindfulness is often described as purposeful attention in the present moment that lends itself to a shift in awareness. This is the basis of self-regulatory techniques in general. In yoga there is the added help of physiological exercises to help the nervous system move more surely toward those changes. Yoga includes more of the body, which provides support for the mindful changes that are being sought. While these two philosophies are organized differently, they both have a clear and parallel intent and various overlapping similarities in practice.

It was Ganesh Baba's belief that the Buddhist path as it was available to westerners was not well suited for our particular cultural needs and more active forms of Self-Realization techniques were needed. His opinion at the time was that the 1970s–'80s version of Buddhist meditation available to the West was aggravating individual psychological "neuroses." It did not provide an adequate structure that individuals could follow without perhaps getting lost in the mind along the way. Since that time most mindfulness programs in the West have included more of a body component to that work.

What Kriya yoga gives us is a fast track to touching divinity, cultivating relationship with Spirit, and understanding Ultimate Universal Unity, or U3 (see box on page 6), in such a way that we can easily experience ourselves belonging to it. This is not to say that an individual cannot be motivated by the equanimity that can come about from any reflective process, but it may not be enough to move the individual forward. Ultimately, it should be understood that the deep work of meditation, which is outlined very nicely in Buddhist texts, only begins to occur once deeper levels of mindfulness and contemplation are arrived at. The practice of Kriya yoga has the capacity to provide the foundation needed to achieve this. We may call upon this wisdom as an initiator for the moral and ethical evolution of our humanity, something deeply needed both socially and culturally at this time.

· · · · · · · · · · · · · · · · · · · · · · · · · · · · · · · · · · · · · · · · · ·

## A Word on Terminology

Throughout this book, we will use many terms to relay the meaning of the word *God*, which some now consider "outdated." Ultimate Universal Unity, or U3, as we shall refer to it, is one of them. Other terms we will use that refer to this concept are Consciousness (or Cosmic Consciousness) with a capital *C* and Spirit with a capital *S*. Other words we will use include Divine, Absolute, and Infinite. In addition Intelligence and Knowledge will both be capitalized when referring to the Knowledge of Self-Realization and the Cosmic Intelligence of Nature, which is the prime creating principle of Nature as shown in the Cycle of Synthesis (see page 59). Occasionally, the word *God* is also used in a quote or a particular reference. In general, these terms are referring to the Ultimate Nondual Energetic Essence from which all that we know has arisen.

There is some differentiation between the expression of U3 and Mother Nature (or simply Nature), the creative force behind the world in which we live, and that of Spirit, or Ultimate Awareness. As will be discussed elsewhere in detail, Kriya yoga is about bringing together the unity of Nature and Spirit to experience the nondual U3 that is discussed in scriptures of all sorts.

Note that while the capitalized version of Nature refers to the ultimate force of Creation, the lowercased form—nature—describes the natural world. We will also use the capitalized version of Self to differentiate the Realized Self from the personal ego-focused self (lowercased).

· · · · · · · · · · · · · · · · · · · · · · · · · · · · · · · · · · · · · · · · · ·

In the West, there has been little focus on internal development, as most of the focus is on external stimuli, "happiness," and material success. We have put cognitive and material expansion above spiritual growth to the detriment of the environment and social relationships. Yet it has come with little promise of increased happiness or contentment. Ganesh Baba saw that the first step toward a spiritualized society was one that led us to evolve enough to realize ourselves as united and connected to everyone and everything and to experience the embodiment of "consciousness" in the largest sense, with a deep acceptance, joy, equanimity, peacefulness, integration, desirelessness, contentment, and compassion. This type of life-changing experience can be brought about in a predictable fashion by following the few simple exercises contained in Kriya yoga as described in this book.

Each path in our history contains within it truths that move humanity's consciousness forward. Each path has relied upon the ones that came before it for its development. As we determine which ones resonate most readily with us, we become more capable of enlightened joy. The joy that is referred to here is not just one of "happiness," which is often situational and therefore transient, but the joy of the deep unconditional love for all beings. The complete interconnectedness of the whole becomes thoroughly visible and the personal experience of reality is transformed. Maya, the veil of duality, is lifted and life beyond illusion becomes accessible.

The task then is to be in this world and also integrate the experience of transcendence. We cannot all retreat to a cave to deeply contemplate the interactions of society and hope that we will propagate internal transformation. Evolution is an active process of engagement with the world. Transformation is a process of Self-Realization and requires a commitment to becoming whole. We have within our future the ability to experience ultimate Truth, ease great suffering, and move toward Self-Realization on this plane during one's lifetime. Self-Realization is the development of insight and direct Knowledge, which becomes the experience of an individual's relationship with the greater whole in the broadest definition imaginable.

. . . . . . . . . . . . . . . . . . . . . . . . . . . . . . . . . . . . . . . . . . . . .

### Maya

The word *Maya* represents illusion; something that is not true reality. The assumption is that there are many ways of perceiving reality, some of which are based in imagination. It doesn't necessarily describe something that isn't there; rather this term as it is used in Indian philosophy refers to another way of understanding the complexities of the human experience. We use the term in reference to a nonduality point of view.

To illustrate the concept of Maya we may look to the *Wizard of Oz*.

In the story, we are introduced to Dorothy, who lives with her aunt and uncle. When her dog Toto's life is threatened, Dorothy runs away from home. She happens upon a fortune-teller who tells her to go back home. In her attempt to return she and Toto are caught in a tornado and become lost in Munchkinland. The challenge for Dorothy is to discern Maya—the dream or illusion—from her reality. She is sent on a quest in the search for Truth. Through her connection with the Tinman, the Cowardly Lion, and Scarecrow, she is faced with parts of herself that she must contend with. The dream begins not as a dream, but as a reality whereby she is knocked unconscious and becomes lost in an unfamiliar world. She, Toto, and her traveling companions become distracted by the many obstacles they must overcome to get to the Wizard of Oz, a master they are told who can help them achieve their deepest desires. Dorothy wants to return home, Tinman wants a heart, Cowardly Lion wants courage, and Scarecrow wants a brain. Led by their desires and engrossed in the search for the great Oz, they put themselves in danger. When they finally find the Wizard of Oz, they are met with an image of power that invokes fear and awe. However, when Toto pulls back the curtain, they discover that the great Oz is nothing more than another illusion, just a projected talking head.

When each character—or aspect of self—is realized, it becomes clear that the answers to the deepest questions reside within. As each character struggles with their desires, they come to see that they possess within them the power to return home, feel courageous, act with compassion, and think independently. Toto represented a small voice that guided the way, leapt out of the reach of danger, demonstrated fearlessness in the face of death, and saw past the veil of Maya. Toto may well be the voice of Dorothy's inner nature. Ultimately, it is Nature that returns us to Spirit and allows for Self-Realization to occur. From the duality of Maya represented in her dream, Dorothy was led on a fantastical adventure to discover and rediscover her way back "home" to the Truth that is and was always within.

· · · · · · · · · · · · · · · · · · · · · · · · · · · · · · · · · · · · · · · · · · · · · · · · · · · ·

## BABAJI AND THE KRIYA LINEAGE

The techniques and knowledge—the science and art of Kriya yoga—have been handed down by the grace of a long lineage, the most recent exponent of which is Ganesh Baba. Kriya yoga as discussed here is a synthesis of many teachings and teachers, but the story of Kriya stems primarily from the roots of one living tree of knowledge (see the lineage chart in figure I.2 below).

# Kriya Lineage
### with Yoga and Naga Roots

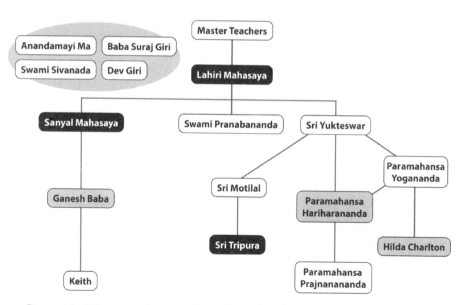

Figure I.2. Kriya yoga lineage chart. Ganesh Baba's teachers are shown with a black background and include Lahiri Mahasaya, Sanyal Mahasaya, and Sri Tripura. See text for descriptions of others in this lineage.

The modern version of Kriya yoga began its dissemination through the work of Lahiri Mahasaya, who brought forth the ancient practice after it had been held in the Himalayas for a long period of time. Lahiri's deep desire, intention, and inspiration brought him to the foothills of the Himalayas where he met his teacher Mahavatar Babaji. This story is told in the *Autobiography of a Yogi* by Paramahansa Yogananda.

Babaji represents a nodal point of communication between humans and Cosmic Consciousness, or U3. The figure of Babaji as depicted in the Kriya yoga line is there as a focal point for those who resonate with a figurative representation. In the story of Kriya yoga, there is no disputing that Lahiri Mahasaya met Babaji in the foothills of the Himalayas, but like any scripture it has to be understood in context. The Himalayan area is a well-known treasure trove of Self-Realized masters. Babaji represents Lahiri Mahasaya's teacher, but more importantly that conglomerate of highly realized beings currently living in their physical bodies in that region. Lahiri Mahasaya is an example of someone connecting with an advanced realized yogi and bringing these teachings off the mountain and back into society for others to learn. At the same time, Babaji provides an example of one that needs no body as they have ascended to a plane where they are teaching all souls at all times. After all, once a Self-Realized master is no longer in their body they become one with the Absolute and are a force for spreading the Knowledge of love, compassion, and wisdom to all who will listen.

As far as we can tell, humans are the only animals that are self-aware to a point of self-reflection and transcendence. Part of our journey here is to learn how to communicate with these realms that have been written about for millennia by the sages and seers of all religions and spiritual pursuits. Some will say that this type of thinking is a delusion but then it must be a mass delusion as many people have connected to Spirit and Nature in this way for millennia despite the fact that our language limits our descriptions of these more ethereal levels of connection. How is it that one can go to church and "speak" with Christ but when the same message comes through in the woods to an individual, they are thought to be hallucinating? Wake up, wake up, wake up! Nature and Spirit are within you and around you.

The world of a human being includes the spiritual, and it is not only a category to list and discuss in philosophy class or read about in Sunday school. The spiritual is a state of being to embrace, explore, and embody, for what it has to offer is the experience of Self-Realization.

If one chooses to pursue a spiritual path there can become less of a need for such figurative representations as Babaji, for the great abstraction of the Absolute simultaneously has everything and nothing within it. That said, a figurative representation of God or Cosmic Consciousness is very helpful to some. The ideal of Babaji in many forms has existed for all time and transcends all creed, race, sex, religion, language, or socioeconomic class. Once the nodal points are connected there is access to Cosmic Consciousness and all the Babajis that ever were are available and in any language or form that is familiar and recognizable to the individual soul who is tapping on the door of the greater Soul. It is this "Soul" that Paramahamsa Hariharananda refers to as "Soul Culture." As he has said, "The Soul and the breath were there before Rama, Krishna, Buddha, Moses, Christ, Mohammed, etc." The Soul is the Soul as the Spirit is the Spirit and Nature is Nature. These are all attempts to use words to describe U3. Rejoice and breathe, feel the joy. This is your life.

The energetic presence of Babaji existed before humans and will exist after humans are gone, as it is the universal Cosmic Consciousness. Babaji is a representation of the essence of Nature touching Spirit. In Kriya yoga it is the physical techniques that adjust one's physiology so that the reception of the essence of all that Babaji represents can come through in a clear and unadulterated fashion. It is through the practice of Kriya yoga, or similar contemplative arts, that we can bring about the deep physiological shift that allows perception of the more subtle and often hidden aspects of our human spiritual experience.

## Masters in the Kriya lineage who passed Kriya on to Ganesh Baba and Keith Lowenstein

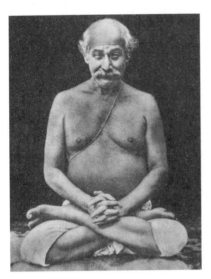

Figure I.3. Lahiri Mahasaya (September 30, 1828–September 26, 1895). Introduced Kriya yoga to the modern world after learning it from his teacher, Babaji.

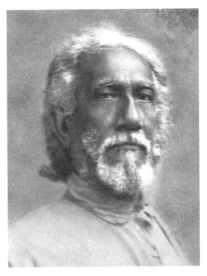

Figure I.4. Sri Yukteswar (May 10, 1855–March 9, 1936). A disciple of Lahiri Mahasaya.

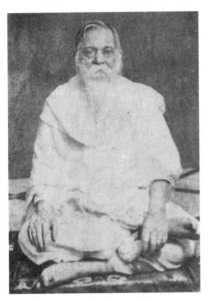

Figure I.5. Sanyal Mahasaya (January 20, 1877–January 18, 1962). A disciple of Lahiri Mahasaya. (Image from the altar Ganesh Baba maintained.)

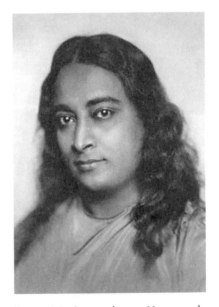

Figure I.6. Paramahansa Yogananda (January 5, 1893–March 7, 1952). A disciple of Sri Yukteswar.

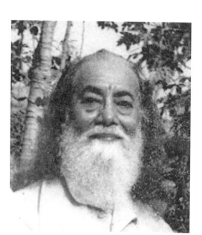

Figure I.7. Paramahamsa
Hariharananda (May 27, 1907–
December 3, 2002).
A disciple of Sri Yukteswar.
(Photo by Mikele34/CC BY-SA.)

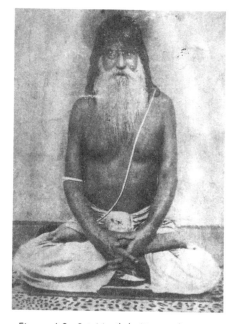

Figure I.8. Sri Motilal. (December 30,
1866–October 10, 1945). A disciple
of Sri Yukteswar. (Image from the altar
Ganesh Baba maintained.)

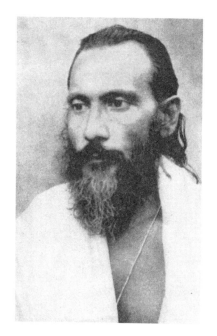

Figure I.9. Sri Tripura. (May 22,
1906–February 8, 1982. A disciple of
Sri Motilal. (Photo by Joy Guru.)

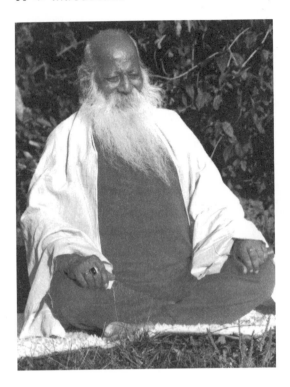

Figure I.10. Ganesh Baba (circa 1892/4–November 19, 1987). Disciple of Lahiri Mahasaya, Sanyal Mahasaya, and Sri Tripura. (Photo by Michelle Cruzel.)

Figure I.11. Paramahamsa Prajnanananda. (August 10, 1959–Present). A disciple of Paramahamsa Hariharananda and current spiritual head of Hariharananda's organizations.

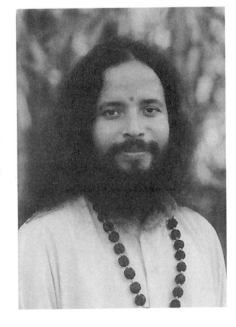

Babaji is neither Hindu nor Christian nor male or female but the nodal point between Nature and Spirit, the prime polarities that together are united in the nondual reality of U3. This is another example that describes Nature (the feminine principle) connecting the life force of the breath to Spirit (the masculine principle) in all its glory of awareness and providing that ultimate connection for an individual. Babaji, in whatever form, will manifest as needed so that the individual self can recognize the Universal/Cosmic Self in order to enter the path and move along on one's journey back to the Absolute.

Lahiri Mahasaya taught Kriya to many students, and Ganesh Baba was one who received his blessing. Ganesh Baba's initial contact with Lahiri Mahasaya was when he was a young child and continued later in life with Lahiri Mahasaya's disciple, Sanyal Mahasaya (Bhupendranath Sanyal). His final Kriya instruction was from by Sri Tripura (Tripura Charan Devsharma), whose instruction was passed down through Sri Yukteswar via Sri Motilal (Sri Motilal Mukhopadhaya).

The teachings you find here are a product of multiple lineages based in Kriya yoga; Advaita Vedanta, a nondualist Indian philosophy; the Bhagavad Gita; and Patanjali's *Yoga Sutras,* which describes the philosophy and practice of yoga and is the root of raja yoga. In addition, Sri Aurobindo—whose work is often referred to as "the yoga of synthesis"—was also influential in Ganesh Baba's studies. Sri Aurobindo's work is another modern interpretation of Advaita Vedanta philosophy, which is traced back to the oldest Upanishads

Approximately 1,000 years ago, a young man named Shankaracharya helped consolidate Advaita Vedanta thought and propagated it throughout India, leaving centers of learning in all the corners of the subcontinent. Shankaracharya started the Dashanami Sanyasi as ten monastic groups. Shri Taponidhi Anand Akhara is one of the affiliated monastic Naga groups. Ganesh Baba belonged to this akhara, which is associated with Shiva and based in Bareilly. Ganesh Baba's teacher in this akhara was Suraj Giri. Later, Ganesh Baba held the position of head monk, a Sri Mahant of this Shaivite Naga akhara (formal association) of Sanyasis and after that Dev Giri took over the role. Ganesh Baba had many other teachers, one of whom was Swami Sivananda, whose organization, the Divine Life Society, provided his initial formal yoga instruction as it did to many of the great yoga teachers of the last hundred years. In addition, Ganesh Baba served as a logistics coordinator for Anandamayi Ma's (see fig. I.12) large ashram in Benares, feeding thousands of people a day. Although Anandamayi Ma was not in this Kriya line she is included here as she was a prominent figure in Ganesh Baba's life. It is Swami Sivananda with whom Ganesh Baba initially became a swami, renouncing his former identity, and thus receiving the title, Ganeshanand Saraswati. Saraswati referring to one who is a highly knowledgeable scholar. Later, when he joined the Shaivite Naga akhara, he then received the title Giri, which refers to those of the forest and those that are warriors. During the years I knew him he went by Sri Mahant Swami Ganeshanand Giri.

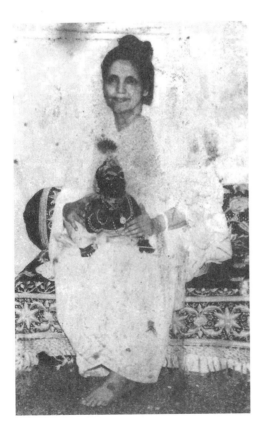

Figure I.12. Anandamayi Ma (April 30, 1896–August 27, 1982). A contemporary of Ganesh Baba and known as a Bengali Saint. She was described by Sivananda Saraswati (of the Divine Life Society) as "the most perfect flower the Indian soil has produced."[1] (Image from the altar Ganesh Baba maintained.)

And while Nagas are typically recognized as fierce warriors rather than intellectuals, Ganesh Baba proved to be both, especially in his sadhana (spiritual practice), for he was also a Kriya yogi in the Lahiri lineage. Ganesh Baba had many other teachers, and their full power remains in every teaching that was passed down to him, as well as their students and their students' students.

I had the rare fortune to be Ganesh Baba's student as a young adult, and also received direct instruction from Paramahamsa Hariharananda during the same time. It just so happens that the lines of Kriya I have been exposed to are all from disciples of Lahiri that are described in *Autobiography of a Yoga* by Paramahansa Yogananda. While preparing this book I had the opportunity to meet, speak, and practice Kriya with Paramahamsa Prajnanananda whom Swami Hariharanada appointed to continue his lineage. Paramahamsa Prajnanananda embodies all that is wonderful in Kriya. In recent years I was also able to speak with and experience the teaching of Swami Pranabananada through his student's student Sri Mukherjee. At nineteen years of age I had early exposure to the power of Hilda Charlton, a disciple of both Paramahansa Yogananda in the 1940s and Nityananda in the 1950s. I have traveled to pay my respects to other members of the Kriya line, and I feel honored to have had the opportunity to meet other spiritual masters including Swami Satchidananda, Pir Vilayat Inayat-Khan, Roy Eugene Davis, Ellen Grace O'Brian, Swami Kriyananda, and Rabbi Gelberman, among others. Some of these meetings were more formal and others included very direct instruction.

This broad exposure to the various interpretations of Lahiri's Kriya superimposed on a very solid base provided by Ganesh Baba and forty years of practice has allowed me to obtain deeper insights into some of the finer practices of Kriya. It is my hope that you may find this Kriya path to be illuminating and life-changing, as so many who have come before us worked diligently to keep it alive.

This book has been written to express deep heartfelt gratitude for the tradition of passing on teachings from generation to generation but also to help provide, as much as possible, a clear and concise guide to these techniques. Each teaching in its own way is unique; it has been experienced, taught, and passed on by individuals, in a particular lineage, who all have their own personal experience with it. The information contained here is an attempt to pass on one particular synthesis of teachings as experienced by one individual schooled in the arts and sciences in the twentieth and twenty-first centuries. Grace alone is in charge from this point forward. May these writings find those who may be looking for them. We believe that ultimately the teacher is within but as the journey proceeds there are fellow travelers who will appear to provide assistance along the way.

*Stretch, extend, and breathe.*
*Become best friends with your breath.*

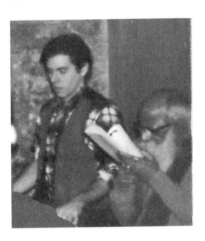

Figure I.13. The author with Ganesh Baba, circa 1982.

# PART I
. . . . . . . . . .
# THE SPIRITUAL AND SCIENTIFIC LINEAGE OF KRIYA

# 1

# Meditation
## *A Contemplative Art*

*Meditation is an emergent property of human experience.*

Siddhartha Gautama sat against the tree feeling the rough bark through his garments. It was a particularly warm day, and the flies were constantly nosing in around his eyes and corners of his mouth. It was proving difficult to focus on the slow pull of his breath, in and out, exhaling until his body became a hollow vessel, then letting the rush of sweet oxygen fill him once again. Today was not like other days. His mind wrestled with him, adamant about its freedom to wallow in the ways sitting was not working out, and how meditating and even breathing were not easy with so many distractions. But he had come here to this tree to do exactly those things: sit, meditate, and breathe. Having left his family behind to pursue the higher wisdom of enlightenment, he now wondered if a renunciant life was truly the most beneficial option. He had walked away from his daily responsibilities to seek higher truth and perhaps in doing so forgot the simplest forms of it.

As he sat against the tree, heat drawing water from his skin, thinking the flies might drive him mad, he refocused his mind on breathing. Believing that the mind is the seat of suffering, he relaxed into a sense of calm and sat up a little straighter, determined to have something to offer this world. This day was not the end of his trials, yet he did not waiver in his fortitude and commitment to better understand the pursuit of peace.

As the story goes, Buddha sat and meditated for many days without food, water, or company, seeking deeper awareness. Perhaps it is because of this day and the many days, months, and years that followed we have the Buddhist tradition of meditation. We can never truly know the journey of the Buddha. What we can gather, however, is that meditation is a practice that one must pursue with passion, perseverance, and dedication.

## A FIRST LOOK AT MEDITATION

Meditation is found among many of the world's traditions and has been practiced since antiquity as an inner art and science of mindful explorations within. Society is most familiar with Eastern traditions of meditation as put forth by Buddhism and yoga; however, most religious faiths have long histories of meditative methods.

Why one chooses to pursue meditation as a practice is rooted in its multitude of benefits. The motivation to devote time and thought toward one's faith is akin to the effort and energy required to better understand oneself. This is the primary benefit of spending time alone with one's breath. Meditation is a practice of adjusting the mind for the attainment of a state of consciousness that is unlike the normal waking state we are used to. While meditation is not in itself a religion or faith, it can be used as a devotional practice, inspiring connection with a unified source such as God and Goddess, or Spirit and Nature as well as Self. It is considered by leaders and masters of meditation to be a precise science, and it follows a particular order that produces clear results. It has structure, principles, and a process that can be repeated and verified. It is also an art unique to the individual, who has some creative license to pursue it in a way that best supports personal growth.

The purpose of meditation is best described as a means to comprehend all levels of ourselves and experience the depth of consciousness within. It is an inwardly guided focus that invites personal transformation on all levels of the human being: physical, biological, psychological, and spiritual.

From our earliest moments we are educated and groomed to think a certain way. We are taught how to examine the world and then how to make judgments in order to verify what we examine. The option to seek answers within our own truths, to ask ourselves for the answers and rely on that as guidance is rarely presented through education. For this reason, many of us remain strangers to ourselves. Very little of our education teaches us how to cultivate the mind much less discipline it. Meditation is truly the only method of developing the mind and harnessing its potential. Through a simple practice we can begin to reclaim our wholeness and our vitality and explore our deeper connection to others.

The human mind (self or ego) can be unruly and antagonistic, undermining our progress, distracting us, keeping us off balance. It may feel as though it holds us emotionally hostage. The mind resists attempts to guide it while it challenges us at every step. However, if we can find stillness, the mind moves aside as we experience more enlightened states of awareness. A still mind is less prone to fantasies, illusions, and distortions. The diligent practice of refocusing, reclarifying, and observing the chaotic chatter of the mind through breath aids the cultivation of a meaningful relationship with oneself.

Another benefit of meditation is that it decreases a sense of anxiety and depression and shows us the underpinnings of these disturbances to help us to better adjust and resolve them. It can also lead us to a greater state of inner balance and stability, offer insight regarding self-sabotaging behaviors, and reduce emotional reactivity. It is tempting to avoid ourselves because it is challenging to address those patterns we don't wish to see, but by becoming more aware of habits and unproductive patterns, we bring them to the forefront and are better able to engage them with our full attention and thus gain control over the mind. This is what we must do to achieve balance in our daily lives.

Although the Buddha was born into royalty and wanted for nothing, he still suffered from being human and was pulled by an inner turbulence to gain more knowledge. And by doing so, he left a legacy, a gift to the world: the insight he cultivated from the likely training he received with master yoga meditators. Buddha is described as seeing meditation as divided into two forms: one-pointed and mindfulness, or insight oriented.[1] One-pointed meditation is an entry place to learn concentration. It usually consists of focusing on a sound, a visual object, or the breath as a way to harness and utilize mindful concentration. Insight-oriented meditation goes deeper and is similar to the latter states of yoga meditation where a goal becomes what is referred to as Liberation, Self-Realization, Truth, or Knowledge. Both require the practitioner to build upon one's self-awareness with focused meditation and routine dedication.

Kriya yoga is a useful mindfulness practice that may initially be more accessible to westerners because it is more somatic (body) focused and action based. In a culture where cognition tends to be overvalued, it is more sensible to begin with a body-mind practice and deepen the somatic experience of meditation over time. Perhaps this is why Buddhism as a mindfulness practice as taught in the West can resonate well with intellectually minded individuals who may struggle with some of the body aspects of other forms. Regardless where one begins their mindfulness practice, both mindful awareness and yoga lead to increasing self-mastery.

Becoming more mindful of the breath and posture can be a very helpful self-regulatory technique and works well for many medical and psychiatric challenges. This is because it has direct effects on the autonomic nervous system and is an entry point for individuals seeking a simple form of physiological relaxation, which can lead to meditation. In the field of mental health, mindfulness has been used to help individuals who struggle with emotions to develop a new relationship with themselves in both body and mind. The introductory breathwork focus of mindfulness helps people to practice mediating reactions through greater understanding of their own emotional control. Learning how to maintain a relaxed and reposed state will nourish new possibilities in one's life and help rewire reactivity.

Through the simple exercises of Kriya yoga one will attain both the mindful awareness of meditation as well as body-based experience of joy. It can be an accelerated path that allows individuals to achieve a deeply embodied sense of Spirit rather quickly. It has the ability to alter the psychological wiring and worldview of the practitioner so that one may experience and understand unconditional love, trust, and integrity. The experience tends to be life changing without needing to be associated with a particular dogma or belief system. It is the task of our time to seek a path of deep contemplation, to interact with society by engaging compassion. We all strive for connection and through this we may change the conversations we have about humanity and help ease the suffering. We yearn for an undiscovered peace, and Kriya outlines a clear path toward our collective evolution and recognition of the Self.

A true desire to experience an awareness outside of the normal waking state will give more power to the quest and is at the heart of every student seeking higher truths. Intention is an essential step in the push toward experiencing oneself from a universal perspective. Faith, devotion, and compassion are all potent tools that assist in becoming anchored to the daily practice even before it produces results beyond mild relaxation. Gratitude, humility, and service become infinite returns within themselves. Of course, we may enrich our lives as well by spending time in nature, exploring movement, studying to exercise the mind, and appreciating art, poetry, music, dance, and literature. For as long as humans have walked the earth, we have possessed the consciousness and curiosity to expand our horizons. We may choose to leave our paths up to fate or we can guide ourselves and each other toward U3 with the structure of Kriya as our compass.

## BEGINNING TO MEDITATE

It is common for a beginning meditation or mindfulness class to use the breath as an initial mindful focal point. There is typically a request to sit up straight, but no additional elaboration on what that means. This is unfortunate and leaves many meditators hunched, often in discomfort if not pain, during years of sitting practice.

The Kriya yoga mindfulness exercise given below includes the breath but its primary focus is on physical posture. In fact, it is the physical posture of one's spine that is of primary importance in Kriya yoga. It is likely that it was also a primary focus in Buddhist meditation as well, as every statue of Buddha portrays him with a divinely straight spine. This is not typically noticed when you look at a statue of Buddha, Ganesh, or Shiva from the front, but is obvious if one glances at a statue from the side.

For any contemplative practice it is essential to develop the ability to sit in a straight upright posture that is comfortable as well as stable and does not cause particular stress or strain on your body or mind. This does require some work. We will begin here with reviewing some of the basics of posture, then move into an exercise to help increase awareness of the spinal column, which functions best anatomically if it is maintained as a finely balanced column and not an arch.

The basic idea is to maintain a bolt upright spine that is both relaxed and supple yet strong and able to sustain you comfortably without movement during a meditative process (see figure 1.1). Ultimately

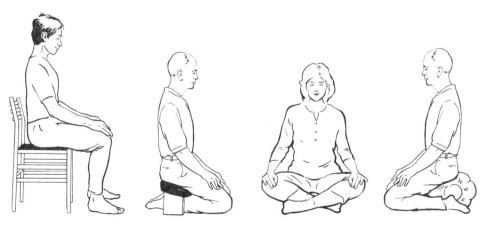

Figure 1.1. Stable posture in various seated positions. Please note the straight spine with the shoulders back and balanced over the pelvis.

meditation is about stillness. Stillness of posture/body, stillness of breath, stillness of mind, and awareness and eventual merging with the vast stillness of Spirit.

Most westerners do better with a pillow placed under their buttocks if they're going to sit on the floor. The goal is to establish a solid pelvic base from which your spine can rise up. Of course, sitting on a chair is also fine but your spine should be maintained upright, not leaning back against the chair. It is fine to move your sacrum toward the back of a firm chair but then you should be sitting straight and tall, which will move most your spine away from the back of almost all chairs.

There will be further discussion regarding refining various aspects of posture in later chapters. Right now the goal is to sit upright and begin with some mindful awareness of breath.

## ⫸ Basic Breathing Exercise

1. Find a comfortable position and turn your attention inward. Once you have arrived at a solid posture, move into a deep, full, relaxed respiration, while maintaining a straight spine. As the breath rises and falls in and out of your body, be mindful of the movement of your chest expanding and rising as you inhale and then relaxing as you exhale.

2. With the next deep breath, allow your shoulders to go up and back. Then, on the exhale, allow them to drop. Spend a few minutes being mindful of this process.

3. Be mindful of your spine from the tip of your coccyx to the top of your skull. Notice if your body is swaying or still. Are you aware of movement in your ribs? If you are seated in a chair, your rib movement should not be constricted by touching the back of a chair. Be mindful of your attention. At this point in time you want to be focused on the breath, the body, the chest, the abdomen, or some other part that is capturing your attention as you maintain a straight and relaxed spine. Be mindful of where your attention goes. If it wanders, bring it back to the task at hand: your breath as one with your posture.

4. As you move into a deeper awareness of the in and out flow of the

breath, gently bring your attention to the uppermost point of your skull. For the next few breaths, see if you can grow a little taller from the vertex of your skull with each inhalation, while staying balanced and secure in the stable base that you have established in your pelvis and its connection to the earth below.

5. Now spend a few minutes being mindful of any of the processes we have just touched on. Being mindful of your breath while at the same time maintaining your posture, being mindful of your posture while at the same time being aware of your breath. This is the foundation of Kriya yoga and can function as the underlying structure for any contemplative practice.

This mindful exercise on posture is presented at the beginning of the book in the hopes that you will maintain a similar awareness of posture while reading it. Maintaining an upright posture with a full, regular, and reposed respiration will allow a greater sense of engagement with the material. Hopefully there will be moments of deeper reflection, where the written material can become an embodied experience, thus infusing some of the spirit of Kriya yoga in the moment.

# 2

# Roots and Fundamentals of Kriya Yoga

*If one maintains correct anatomical posture, all else will come.*
GANESH BABA

Kriya yoga and many other oral contemplative traditions have been passed down from teacher to student for millennia and have been offered in various flavors around the globe. The earlier forms of this type of meditative practice likely go back five thousand years or more, and some believe that meditative practices such as Kriya yoga have been in existence for over ten thousand years. As civilizations developed and became more "modern," esoteric and spiritual practices were often kept out of sight if not entirely hidden. As civilization evolved, education became ever more specialized and often neglected more traditional practices. Throughout the past few thousand years, practices that contributed to Self-Realization were often banned or restricted due to the potential political ramifications for those "in power."

While it does appear those who knocked on the Kriya yoga door were most often welcomed, this was not the case in other traditions, which were curated and protected by a privileged and segregated community that prevented the so-called lower castes and outcastes in India from accessing the teachings. Women, too, were often forbidden to enter these traditions even though many of the traditions held Mother Nature—the divine feminine principle and the source of all Creation—to be most sacred. This is easily seen in the practices of yoga and tantra throughout India that focus on the divine Nature of the feminine.

In fact, it is the creative power of Mother Nature, the Divine Mother that is woven into many of the Kriya lines. Although this is not widely known Mother Nature, the Divine Mother, is often the initial attraction for those who enter the Kriya line. An important point that Ganesh Baba imparted to those he taught was, "One can only truly know the father (Spirit) by first knowing the mother (Nature)." In the case of Ganesh Baba his personal association with the divine feminine principle was most evident through his service to Anandamayi Ma and his devotion to the Divine Mother (Nature) in all her manifestations.

Despite their secretive nature and exclusion of women, contemplative practices spread, allowing for the development of rich traditions and cross-fertilization throughout the many subcultures in India and across Asia.

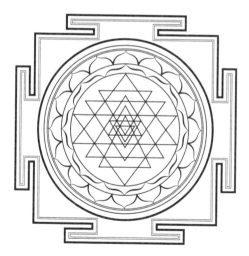

Figure 2.1. The Sri Yantra is often associated with Goddess-focused spiritual paths in India. It is used in meditation as a visual representation of Cosmic Consciousness. The Sri Yantra symbol is a visual equivalent of Om, the primordial nodal vibration. The Cycle of Synthesis, which will be discussed later in the book, is a conceptual representation of this abstract yantra. They represent the nondual union of Spirit and Nature while at the same time reflecting all its potential manifestations. The pinnacle of Self-Realization.

As these techniques became infused by the practices of the Middle East, Persia, China, Tibet, and Nepal as well as Japan, Indochina, and others, they became richly multicultural and adorned with new perspectives.

Religions such as Judaism, Islam, Christianity, Zoroastrianism, Jainism, Buddhism, and Hinduism also played a significant part in the development of such wisdom traditions, and many faith-based organizations around the world promoted a variety of contemplative practices. Some of these practices remain alive and vibrant today, continuing to bring joy, transforming the religion from within, and supporting it from generation to generation. Unfortunately, some have lost their sense of aliveness and therefore attractiveness to younger generations, as the practices themselves became rigid, dry, and brittle. It is of utmost importance that young people are able to reinterpret and continually reintroduce these practices in the language and spirit of the times in which they live. Of course, this does not mean ignoring the past but rather simply and tenderly preserving it while allowing it evolve and be transmuted.

Yoga, and Kriya yoga specifically, is one such adaptable practice. Certain specific roots of Kriya yoga can be traced in the disciplines of raja yoga (referring to the royal path), karma yoga (emphasizing action or service), bhakti yoga (emphasizing devotion), kundalini yoga (focusing on sound and mantra), jnana yoga (emphasizing knowledge), and hatha yoga (focusing on physical techniques). Kriya takes its philosophical nourishment from the Yoga Sutras of Patanjali, the Vedas, and especially the Bhagavad Gita, and then synthesizes these ancient practices and philosophies with modern-day physics, physiology, and psychology. The Yoga Sutras of Patanjali, written sometime between 200 BCE and 400 CE, is considered to be one of the most thorough treatises on the practice of eight-limbed yoga. We will explore this system in more detail later on in the book.

At its heart, Kriya yoga is a contemplative art that works to develop an individual's fitness in body, mind, and spirit. It teaches integration so that students may cultivate a relationship with one's own self slowly and move toward a personal experience with Spirit that leads ultimately to a deep sense of compassion for all of humanity and the union of Nature and Spirit.

The contemplative arts involve a uniquely creative process and are unlike other forms of art that may tend to limit modes of expression through the structure of words, forms, images, and movements. In the contemplative arts, the practice moves one toward an awareness of the infinite dimensions within the human experience, which occurs as we explore beyond the fourth dimensional space-time continuum currently recognized by science. Kriya is one example of a contemplative art that offers a systematic way of self-exploration of the inner connection between Nature and Spirit within a human being, which is a gateway to the Infinite.

Kriya yoga is also considered a science in that the physiological changes experienced by an individual are reproducible in another individual in a similar state of health. A regular practice of yogic exercises leads to increased proficiency in bringing about these physiological changes, which in turn modulate our mind, body, and spirit to bring about an increased awareness and sensitivity to more subtle energies. This scientific path guides one toward spiritual insight. Its transformative quality is unifying and will aid those who commit to it in achieving their own Self-Realization. Thus, the scientific side of Kriya yoga guides one toward spiritual insight as surely as its creative side allows for rich inner explorations that can last a lifetime.

The word *yoga* means "union" and refers to the union of the body, mind, and spirit. There are many routes and ways to establish this union and even within yoga there are a variety of techniques and philosophies to follow based on what suits a person best. Ultimately, yoga gives a practitioner the ability to suspend ideation at will; that is, to increase their ability to modulate their thoughts, achieve one-pointed concentration, and enter new dimensions of experience.

The longevity of Kriya yoga relies on the richness of experience as well as its flexibility in meeting people where they are with low fuss techniques. Thus, viewing Kriya through the lens of contemplative science is to make it as specific and distilled as possible. This means removing superfluous obstacles, rituals, or any type of connection to a particular belief system, which will hopefully simplify the task for the practitioner. Kriya yoga is about experiencing the unity of Spirit and Nature, and its regular practice leads to the embodiment of that experience, which is Self-Realization.

## THE FUNDAMENTALS OF KRIYA YOGA

Kriya yoga, or simply Kriya, is fundamentally a method that utilizes posture, respiration, visualization, and a repetitive internal or external vocalization (a vibration, so to speak) in a systematic fashion to redirect attention from an outward focus to an inward focus. It is a practice in the retraction of our outwardly focused senses. Used together these exercises lead to changes of the waking conscious state and open up our perception to a world of subtler metaphysical energies that become part of our awareness. Ultimately these explorations lead to insights, joy, and an expanded ability for contemplation. We become part of the all that is, all that ever was, and all that ever will be. As lofty as statements like these may sound, they are often the framework on which spiritual development and exercises are based.

### A Deeper Understanding of Meditation

The word *meditation* has taken hold in contemporary society. We use it in common everyday language, i.e., "let me meditate on that." In English it is related to the word *mediate* and reflects the true work we encounter while doing it. Meditation is, in a way, a mediation between the body, the mind, the conscious, the unconscious, and the supraconscious; in other words the *self,* which in this usage refers to the Freudian model of the id (unconscious drives), the ego (that part most of us think of as our personality), the superego (the moral observer of the id and ego), and *Self,* which equates with the realization of the God within, or Spirit.

The goal of meditation is to remain still between the various aspects of our being and view ourselves more clearly to attain a deeper inner resonance and stillness. In Kriya yoga this is accomplished via a set exercises for each realm of the human experience. It removes the guesswork and accelerates the integration of the whole person. Meditation is a tool that allows us to connect to the energetic body of the earth and the subtle realms of energy, as well as to Nature's Intelligence, which is present in every cell, molecule, subatomic particle, and beyond. It is a practice of "knowing thyself" and becoming more embodied, enriched, and connected to the human experience as a whole. The work of Kriya comprises the physical practice of sitting, breathing, and moving through exercises with persistence, intention, dedication, and curiosity.

We must become clear about what meditation is, since it is the basis of Kriya. Meditation begins with the transition between states of consciousness, particularly when one's awareness shifts from a normal waking state to a state of focused concentration. It is a condition where *emergent properties* (those properties that are not predicted individually by the parts or by the sum of the parts but manifest as result of the parts' interaction within a system) start to take place within the central nervous system altering the brain's perception of itself.* This shift can change a person's perception so that subtle energies, or emergent properties, become tangible and more readily available to interact with, explore, and enjoy. More often than not, the first contact with subtler

---

*The brain can be thought of as a number of different organs that have grown up (evolved) closely together and been forced to learn to get along as they occupy a tightly enclosed space (the skull). Meditation takes the brain as a whole and begins to work with its relative parts, changing the pattern of communication within. This in turn causes new patterns of interaction to occur that we experience as different states of awareness, which allow us to access the more-subtle energy of intuition and more. Our brain and spinal cord provide us with endless varieties of experience as we learn to modulate the inner world toward Self-Realization via an infinite array of emergent properties that spring forth as the central nervous system's patterns of interactions within itself modulate and evolve. Once those shifts in communication occur it is easier to find one's way back, and with practice it becomes part of daily experience. With time, entering states of deep meditation is no different than going to sleep. They are both changes in our state of conscious awareness. It is the learned external and inner action that bring about these changes in a reliable and predictable fashion. Alcohol and drugs can also alter conscious states of awareness and even make us unconscious. The difference here is the use of exogenous molecules that alters our central nervous system versus using our own inner technology to do so. These drug-induced changes can be similar in some ways but are not ultimately the same.

energies is coupled with the feeling of love and an all-encompassing sense of joy. Certainly, perception changes as these emergent properties begin to take over the typical styles of communication within the nervous system. The meditator experiences the communion with Nature and Spirit while being fully present to witness that union.

When the practices of Kriya bring enough stillness to the system, then the bottomless well of creative energy that is Nature rises to meet the evolutionary force of Spirit, and both move toward Source, the Absolute. In this state the duality of normal waking consciousness meets the nonduality of the unstruck sound, or what Ganesh Baba referred to as the U3, the mystical, the sacred, the Word, which is also referred to as the primordial nodal vibration, or *pronov* (historically spelled *pranava* but altered by Ganesh Baba to resonate with the phrase "primordial nodal vibration" and a more English spelling).

Meditative states are not mindless. Our awareness of our conscious mind is still present but the perspective shifts, moving toward a supraconscious state that historically was often referred to as the metaphysical realm. This is not unlike going to sleep, having a dream, or experiencing any other change in one's physiological state brought on by illness, fever, medication, alcohol, recreational drugs, or anesthetic agents. Any change in consciousness also alters perception of time. Meditative states are simply just another place on the spectrum of consciousness as depicted in figure 2.2 on page 35.

Meditation is an exercise that helps us learn how to further direct and change our consciousness. Thinking about consciousness and meditation in this light can be helpful as it provides a reference point to the other states of consciousness that almost everybody has experienced.

Despite the fact that there has been considerable work done since the 1960s on differentiating psychosis from mystical experiences, most notably from such pioneers as Stanislaus Grof, Andrew Newberg, Francis Lu, David Lukoff, Roger Walsh, Ken Wilber, Abraham Maslow, and others, the fields of psychiatry and psychology still struggle with sorting out transcendent experiences. Many of these "ultra or trans" experiences are

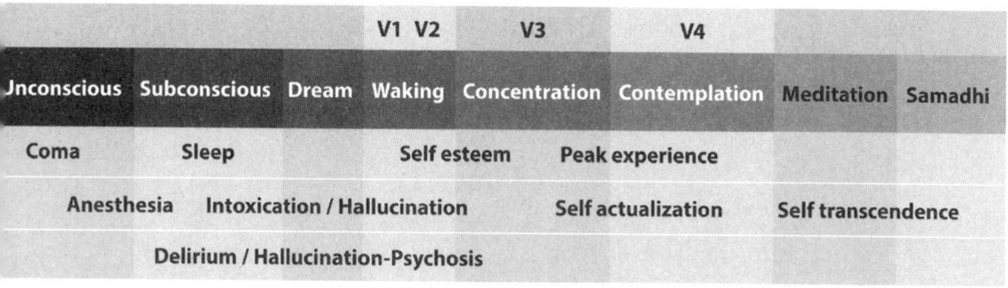

| | | V1 V2 | | V3 | | V4 | | |
|---|---|---|---|---|---|---|---|---|
| Unconscious | Subconscious | Dream | Waking | Concentration | Contemplation | Meditation | Samadhi |
| Coma | Sleep | | Self esteem | | Peak experience | | |
| Anesthesia | Intoxication / Hallucination | | | | Self actualization | | Self transcendence |
| | Delirium / Hallucination-Psychosis | | | | | | |

Figure 2.2. Spectrum of consciousness. This diagram is a depiction of the human experience of awareness or consciousness. V1–V4 are included to show how they relate to our overall awareness within the four initial practices of Kriya, which will be discussed in chapters 4 and 5.

pathologized. Humans are fragile, resilient, and complex creatures capable of both psychosis and spiritual awakening, and it can be challenging to detect the differences between healthy evolutionary experiences and psychotic episodes derived from disordered brain physiology.

One of the fundamental problems is that the field of mental health, as well as society, has yet to fully embrace the idea that transcendent experiences can be a healthy, integrative part of everyday life. That said, psychoses can be very disabling for an individual and attending to them as soon as possible is an important part of Western medicine. In the process, however, we cannot lose track of the fact that not everyone who initially presents to an emergency room with what appears to be an altered mental status and an experience of "oneness" is necessarily psychotic, and vice versa. If in fact they maintain conceptually organized thought processes and have some control over their attention, they may not be psychotic in the traditional sense. Psychoses associated with processes such as schizophrenia typically leave an individual much more disorganized in their thoughts and unable to appreciate their situation in a broader context.

One challenge researchers have in embracing this concept of "normal" transcendental experiences is that a collective understanding of "awakenings" has not yet been organically imbedded within society. Conversations about mental health need to stretch to include a wider swing on the pendulum. With enough space and time, more researchers themselves could become fluent in transcendental states and may then be better equipped to tease out particular nuances in individuals who may be encountering spontaneous awakening and others who may benefit from mental-health treatment.

This is a complex subject that has been written about in great length by others, and therefore will not be elaborated on much further here. It should be noted, however, that although Kriya yoga is a technique that is well suited for rapid advancement of compassion and spiritualization for those who are inclined to move in that direction, it is not suitable for those having difficulties with the spectrum of psychosis.

## Prana

Meditation is the state that invokes our nervous system to begin a holistic integration process, and through it we can begin to perceive the infinite meaning of consciousness and feel that we are directly connected to the life force energy prevalent in all living things. This energy is called prana, and our prana comes from our breath.

Swami Hariharananda was often fond of saying in his classes, "What is upholding your body? Your breath only. But who is pulling the breath? The power of God is pulling the breath. It is why you are alive."[1]

In Kriya yoga, a key element is the exploration and management of the energy and function of prana. Other cultures have terms for prana such as *qi* (*chi*) in Chinese medicine or *ki* in Japanese. Cultures in the Pacific Ocean such as New Zealand, Hawaii, Tahiti, and Polynesia have been found to use the term *mana* to refer to the life-force energy. The Iroquois had a term for the spiritual power in humans, referred to as *Orenda*. In homeopathy, the term *vital force* is used to describe an energy that pervades all living organisms. In Hebrew the words *ruach* and *neshamah* refer to the breath as spirit, and the Greeks used the word *pneuma* in a similar fashion. This concept is fairly common across humanity, but somewhat lacking in acceptance by modern-day Western cultures. This is connected to our lack of acceptance or appreciation for spirituality as a natural part of our everyday lives.

## Matter, Prana, and Spirit

Death arrives when the current of life, the prana, leaves. With death the connection between Spirit and the life force in that particular body is severed. Our individual mind also fades as it is a field that the current of life brings into this existence. That is not to say that the prana of the physical molecules of the body is gone, as it is not. Each molecule returns to the greater environment and continues its dance. It is just the association between these molecules within one living human being that has changed. The Intelligence of Nature, that master organizing energy, continues within the individual atoms and molecules.

The physical body serves as the vehicle that attracts the infusion of prana. When the heart is beating, the brainstem is commanding the respiratory system to draw breath, and when the nervous system is intact, the physical body attracts the life essence, prana, which infuses the physical system with life, an emergent property that is not predictable from the sum total of the physical parts. Similarly, when the physical body fails, meaning it is no longer capable of sustaining life, prana no longer runs through the body, death ensues, as the field of mind can no longer be maintained without the current of life. This is when the individual self/ego whom we identified with a particular body and mind is considered deceased. This explanation of our life energy will be explored again later when we look more deeply at Ganesh Baba's cosmology integration of science and Indian philosophy called the Cycle of Synthesis.

As we enter this world we take our first breath and make our own individual connection with prana. When we leave this world we take our last breath, and the current of life in a body is gone, as prana blends with the greater whole. With states of meditation one begins to learn about prana through experience, and as we learn to use Kriya yoga to control our breath in a systematic, creative, scientific fashion, we learn what our breath's impact is on our physiology and our perceptions.

# 3
# Spirit-Infused Science

*A new kind of [scientific] theory is needed which drops the basic commitments and at most recovers some essential features of the older theories as abstract forms derived from a deeper reality in which what prevails is unbroken wholeness.*

DAVID BOHM, PH.D.,
*WHOLENESS AND THE IMPLICATE ORDER*

What is science if it does not lead us to reconsider the meaning of our world and our relationship to it? There have been a variety of definitions for science and philosophy and various attempts to look at the philosophy of science. It was not too long ago that the disciplines of art, science, philosophy, and religion were interwoven. As the march of science has progressed, the general rubric has been to look at smaller and smaller parts. This promotes a reductionistic aspect of science that unfortunately ripples through the fabric of education and impacts our ability to make more holistically informed decisions. As new branches of science have developed, such as those looking at systems theory, chaos, and the properties of emergence, they have demonstrated that the whole is not necessarily the sum of its parts. We make the argument that areas that are unknown, or are at this point immeasurable by our current dials and meters, be considered as potentially useful as a form of scientific pursuit.

Just because something cannot be measured with the current state of technology does not mean it does not exist. For example, previously invisible microbes, DNA, and subatomic particles were barely elements of imagination in the late 1880s but are now accepted as common knowledge. In 1888 Santiago Ramón y Cajal demonstrated that the nervous system was made up of individual neurons, which he was able to see under a microscope. The further advancement of technology has allowed us to witness activity between neurons in the brain. It is now possible with an fMRI to see the physiological changes that occur with various emotions and observe changes in neuronal activity directly related to emotional responses. Granted, this new cognitive science is still in its infancy, but ten decades ago you would have thought it irrational to imagine there might be machines with the capability of measuring emotion by looking inside one's head and seeing the activity of neurons.

But humanity did not arrive at this point through the use of science only. Intelligence, intuition, persistence, creativity, and curiosity helped humanity progress and develop civilizations comprised of individuals who can work together as a whole and gain collective insights. While Western science attempts to objectify what it studies, a contemplative science such as Kriya attempts to understand and integrate what it observes.

Science is limited by the frame of time, the prevailing paradigm in which a particular scientific view is pursued. This can make it difficult to reflect on and understand one's own cultural biases in the moment. Contemporary slices of time show a technological advance that allows for collective conversations in a way that has never before existed. The advent of the internet now bridges distinct points of view and offers snapshots of vastly different experiences in a short slice of life. It shakes up our current worldview and puts under a magnifying glass what would otherwise be hidden from view. It is from this new paradigm that we must move forward while trying to embrace the disparate domains of our human collective experience as ones that can be better understood from a spiritually-informed scientific standpoint.

Most science is powered by an observation or description of a particular phenomenon. A hypothesis is then made to explain the phenomena and in the core sciences, reflects a pursuit of a causal mechanism or mathematical relationship. The hypothesis then predicts a particular outcome that can ideally be quantitatively measured with additional observations and repeated by others. It is the ability to get observable data by different people in different settings that is the bedrock behind the power of science. Experiments are further devised to test the hypothesis/theories and science inches forward over time as paradigms change due to the results that are found.

Although science has had numerous insights during the past century, there has been a relentless march toward dismissal of what it has found. Often scientific results are misrepresented or confusing or are not clearly understood, but dismissing them for these reasons alone is shortsighted and divisive. Despite the fact that the daily existence of individuals in the West is heavily reliant on science and technology, the current trends to disregard science when it flies in the face of short term political, economic, and religious motivations is slowly eroding rational dialogue.

These days, discussing science, religion, and spirituality together can be quite challenging. Centuries of time have passed, but it does not appear that the debate has gotten much past Copernicus or Galileo. Change is still seen as threatening, and our current town square, the media, is taking liberties to spin its rhetoric from disparate points of view, obscuring logic and rational thought. Intelligent and collective debate has taken a backseat to reactivity. Extraordinary claims that are for or against either spirituality, religion, or science must be looked at objectively and not dismissed merely because one perspective has the bully pulpit at the moment.

It is our challenge as a society to be intellectually curious and dogma avoidant. This outlook can only be cultivated through education and understanding that occurs in the experiential and objective realms. Just as there are physical laws such as gravity, there are physiological patterns preserved among species that interact in ways that are increasingly predictable. How we embrace the synthesis of various worldviews will define us as a species and either allow our evolution to unfold or cause the destruction of the current relative dynamic balance of Mother Nature that we currently enjoy.

## DELUSION OF CONSCIOUSNESS

Albert Einstein, unquestionably one of the greatest scientists in the past few hundred years, had a tremendous influence on the evolution of our understanding of physics and mathematics. He also had a profound impact as a compassionate philosopher, as shown in a letter he wrote in 1949 that was published in an article in the *New York Times* on March 29, 1972. An ordained rabbi had written explaining that he had sought in vain to comfort his nineteen-year-old daughter over the death of her sister, "a sinless, beautiful, 16-year-old child." Einstein wrote back in reply:

> A human being is a part of the whole, called by us "Universe," a part limited in time and space. He experiences himself, his thoughts and feelings as something separated from the rest—a kind of optical delusion of his consciousness. This delusion is a kind of prison for us, restricting us to our personal desires and to affection for a few persons nearest to us. Our task must be to free ourselves from this prison by widening our circle of compassion to embrace all living creatures and the whole nature in its beauty. Nobody is able to achieve this completely, but the striving for such achievement is in itself a part of the liberation and a foundation for inner security.[1]

Currently, humanity is caught in what Einstein called in his letter above, a "delusion of consciousness." Humans are blessed with the rare ability to interact with ideas of self, thoughts, feelings, and yet we perceive it as being separate from the rest of existence. We think of ourselves as the center of our own universe around which all else revolves. The detriment of this type of thinking is that it ultimately restricts us from connecting to an expanded sense of compassion. Moreover, it narrows our view to only those closest to us at best and allows us to withhold compassion for those we choose not to extend understanding to. It further restricts us from embracing our life-giving and sustaining connection to our planet. As Einstein relates, this mental prison is the compound that creates and blocks an even greater worldview. Our task then must be to widen our circles of compassion to embrace even those we do not relate to, to embrace all living creatures, and assume some level of responsibility for the well-being of all sentient creatures, nature, and the universe as a whole. Kriya and other such practices can help us learn how to sublimate hate into love and acceptance.

Reflecting on physicist Werner Heisenberg's uncertainty principle, we know that the observation of a physical phenomenon affects the system being observed. In metaphysical experiences the sages confirm that the same phenomenon holds. Theoretical physicist John A. Wheeler elaborated on Heisenberg's theories when he wrote about the participatory universe:

The universe does not exist, out there, independent of us. We are inescapably involved in bringing about that which appears to be happening. We are not only observers. We are participators. In some strange sense this is a participatory universe.[2]

This correlates with John Bell's theorem in which he states very briefly that "reality is non-local."[3] This has been interpreted to mean that the world we see does not exist until we see it, and it is this act of observing by itself that affects other elementary particles far away. Does this mean the universe itself is alive? That as we live and breathe we create an ever-present, ever-evolving infinite universe that can be observed as well as it can observe? Can we really be independent beings if we are so interrelated, or entangled,* with the actions in our environment from subatomic particles to our most obvious human relationships? These questions in turn lead us to wonder, Can anything really be identified as separate?

America's early environmentalist John Muir is noted to have said that "when we try to pick out anything by itself, we find it hitched to everything else in the universe."[4] The nondual philosophy of Advaita Vedanta mirrors these examples of environmental science and quantum physics. We will see this illustrated again later when we look at Ganesh Baba's Cycle of Synthesis that connects modern physics, evolution, and Indian philosophy.

## SCIENCE, TRUTH, AND A NEW PARADIGM

We are living on a planet in physical bodies—a condition that clearly fosters our belief that we are separate from everything else. And although our bodies are clearly infused by Spirit, we celebrate our physicality almost to the neglect of intelligence, higher mind, and life. We can see the material world, feel physical energies such as heat and cold, move around in three-dimensional space, and measure and watch the fourth dimension of time pass by as we go through life. As we move forward into the realm of more subtle energy, quantitative measurement becomes more difficult. We might measure the electrochemical effects of a physiological processes, but from a scientific view, how might we measure life?

Our language uses phrases like "brought back to life" to describe what happens when those who have ceased to breathe or have a

---

*In broad general terms the quantum mechanics definition of *entanglement* is when one particle is influenced by its environment and in turn influences another particle despite a seeming lack of connection in space.

heartbeat are returned to a waking state. But our current scientific knowledge does not have a "life meter" to definitively determine levels of life within a biological system. Nor do we have a "mind meter." We have only a limited vision of the inner spaces of the human being. An EEG, for example, is a brain meter to some degree but cannot peer into the field of a mind. If we cannot determine what exactly life is or mind is, how might we discuss it in scientific realms?

Cognitive neuroscience is a scientific discipline that is making inroads in this area. In fact, it has shown us that our adult brains can and do grow. Our frontal cortex can get thicker with meditation, and we are capable of making new neurons in the hippocampus, the memory areas of our brains. While even with these new technologies we cannot measure mind in detail, we are beginning to see that mind causes our brain energy/metabolism to change in specific ways, depending on the tasks at hand.

Let us now briefly return to what historically have been considered the core sciences: physics, mathematics, chemistry, and molecular biology. Even in what we consider to be hard science, consensus does not make something true. The defining line between what is truth and what is not truth continues to be eroded by rigidity, fear, and greed.

Bertrand Russell wrote that the goal of science is to "increase precision [of knowledge] without diminishing certainty." He understood that vague knowledge had more likelihood of truth than precise knowledge, but that it was also less useful. We can consider the assimilation of knowledge as taking the shape of a pyramid. The base is a broad collection of data. As we move up to the point of the pyramid, information becomes more precise and the excess or unrelated data, while acting as a foundation for the point of precision and understanding, becomes less relevant. It is difficult to transcend one's own paradigm, but it is increasingly necessary to do so to define knowledge that we can rely on.

Science and truth have often been inextricably coupled, one meaning that the other is absolute. Science is a structured discipline of discovery always giving way to another perspective, a new level of knowledge that adds to the essential components of the data that came before it. When we apply this ideal to contemplation, we have a rich panorama of knowledge that transforms into deep wisdom. In the case of a contemplative art such as Kriya yoga, we are the meter that is experiencing, sensing, and measuring the experimental results of a meditation process in which rigidity and fear are exposed as weakness in the presence of joy and compassion. Hence, with a more integrated science, humans can become more integrated as well. By using intellect symbiotically with the heart we are better able to rise to the potential of what it can mean to be human.

We are pure potential, capable of changing, given new insight or new interaction. It is doubtful that humans will ever reach a state where there are no further questions, where everything is pure factual knowledge. Science informed by a moral and compassionate compass, one that can include emotional intelligence instead of throwing it out, is possibly the best method we currently have. It is a way of moving forward and better understanding the nature of the cosmos in which we live, which lives within us, and from which we act and interact with all that surrounds us in the physical, biological, psychological, and spiritual realms.

We will continue to investigate and reflect on the contemplative sciences from the standpoint of emergent properties. To quote Einstein once again, "The most beautiful experience we can have is the mysterious. It is the fundamental emotion which stands at the cradle of true art and true science."[5] Through the contemplative sciences humanity can move forward and learn how to regularly experience "the mysterious" in ways that broaden and enliven our joy and our understanding of ourselves and each other.

# 4

# Balancing the Basics

---

*Kriya is a foundational practice.*

---

We are all energy, and this guide to the practice of Kriya is a look at the various types of energy and how they are experienced, utilized, modified, generated, received, and transmitted. The energetic forces that we are most familiar with are gravity and electromagnetic energy. Gravity is an independent force that we feel on our bodies all the time. We take it for granted, but if we drop something or fall, we're quickly reminded that gravity is always at play.

Our physical senses help us navigate the physical world, and even before we open our eyes in the morning, we experience light. Light is part of the electromagnetic spectrum and we will use this spectrum of energy to help demonstrate levels of energy that are outside our current ability to measure with machines. However, no electronic device can come close to sensing and integrating the amount of information the human nervous system is capable of. Can all that we experience be reduced down to the interactions of electrical and chemical energies within the three-dimensional confines of our body? Is it all just physiology—the body, the brain, and central nervous system—or is there something else at work?

As previously established, prana in the form of breath is our connection between the physical universe and the space-time continuum that reaches into a more subtle energetic universe, which is beyond what our technology can currently measure. In order to experientially explore prana, we must build a structure to generate and manage this energy in new ways. We do this by using posture and breath. It is the breath that holds the key to the modulation and balance of this energy. As one begins to add additional concentration and energy movement exercises to one's practice, one begins to further change and adjust one's physiology. The perception of the physical world shifts with this exploration of prana as one's practice deepens.

The first breath of life begins with birth and throughout life, breath modulation and focused concentration allow an internal focus on prana, which can be experienced in ever-increasing subtleties. These subtleties are the beginning stages of transcendence that offer insights into the nature of the universe as described for millennia in spiritual scriptures and since the dawn of the 1900s in modern physics. Ultimately, through increasingly finer shifts in one's awareness, the connectedness of all the known and unknown aspects of the Absolute present themselves in perfect harmony.

However, in order to experience and balance these subtleties of energy, we need to sit straight and become a refined antenna through which Spirit may better align with our awareness. We need to pay attention to breath so our system will increase in strength and be able to hold more and more energy as it passes from the unseen realm into this one. Posture and breath, posture and breath, posture and breath. Posture and breath create the ultimate foundation from which this journey begins.

We are breathing life while life is breathing us. The universe came into existence with its own form of respiration, a vibration so to speak. As it says in John 1:1, "In the beginning was the Word, and the Word was with God, and the Word was God." In this vibration, Word or Om (Aum), we have the root of the infinite energetic realities available to human awareness. With more awareness comes more harmony in life, more balance inside and outside the body. As it is internally so it is cosmically. Balance is the pinnacle of existence; all of life tries to be in homeostasis with itself and with its environment.

As a species, humans are fairly resilient and can bounce back from many extremes. We learn to rebound from mishaps, regroup after stressful encounters, and reorganize after wasting precious moments of time. However, if we are to maintain optimal health or move forward on a spiritual path, we must strive for more personal responsibility in our lives. From the moment we are born, coming through the birth canal into the world, we are in a vital and active practice of balance between the forces within the body and those outside. Life requires even the tiniest human form to fight for existence, enhancing the likelihood that our first breath will be victorious. Life and our relationship to it are managed through the ebb and flow of balance from the very first breath to the very last.

Balance first begins to develop in the womb and continues after birth through the natural rhythms transferred from one human being to another. The baby is learning self-regulation during this time. While a baby is dependent and needs to rely on others for protection and food, his nervous system is learning through interaction with caregivers. A caregiver that is relaxed and nonreactive teaches the new baby how to be the same by coregulation. The baby recognizes the mother's breathing patterns whether they are frantic and anxious or confident, smooth, and nurturing. If the household is disruptive and full of chaos, the infant will be less successful in self-regulating toward calm due to the experience of co-dysregulation. When these basic rhythms are disturbed or led by fear or trauma, problems with self-regulation and health develop as well. Challenges with dysregulation become apparent in behavior, emotional outbursts, anger, depression, anxiety, and an inability to learn or assimilate new information.

We are moving into a time where the majority of childhood experience is immersed in trauma. Fewer adults are skilled in ways to cope, and fewer elders are present that can pass on wisdom. Trauma and violence have now become a significant part of everyone's existence whether it is experienced directly, through peers, or through social media channels. It has become clear that young children who have been exposed to trauma have greater difficulty with self-regulation and struggle in society later in life. The solution thus far has been to ostracize kids who are underperforming in school and to build more prisons.

We have become selfish in our interactions with each other and the earth itself. Through the honoring of Mother Nature and her cycles we might learn about how to reorganize our motivations toward self-regulation and ultimately Self-Realization. In seeking balance through breathwork and the continued practice of Kriya, one may also peek into such metaphysical realities and find calmness, clarity, and compassion.

## FINDING BALANCE IN MEDITATION

Many people say that they can't meditate because they can't concentrate. Few people, on the other hand, say they can't drive. Meditation and driving are really very similar (see figure 4.1). Just driving down

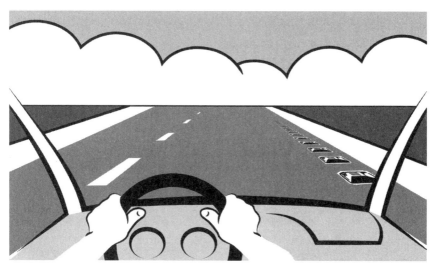

Figure 4.1. Meditation is like driving. Both require a practice of focused attention that is frequently adjusted. Of course, one should never drive and meditate at the same time.

the road requires constant adjustments to speed and direction. Even on a straight road steering needs to be adjusted to keep the automobile in the correct lane and prevent it from driving off the road. Occasionally, if the driver is distracted the car may drift to one side or the other. When this happens, the driver doesn't typically berate herself for not paying attention enough to drive. What the driver does do is to correct for the distraction and continue to move forward.

This is exactly what happens in meditation. Meditation is a practice; it is the practice of attending to the moment. If one begins to daydream or gets caught in a cycle of anxiety-provoking thoughts, one only needs to redirect the thought process back to the posture, breath, third eye, and/or a mantra. It is no different than redirecting the car. You are continuing to move forward and are engaging in the "practice" of meditation. Meditation is an activity of attention training; the greater your ability becomes, the finer you'll be able to focus your attention for longer periods of time.

It is the expertise that develops in these techniques that helps one move down the road toward Self-Realization. So please, please do not be dissuaded when distraction comes. If you cannot focus for even a few minutes at a time, remember this is a practice, a journey that begins with first steps. One is almost certain to feel somewhat unsteady at first and have difficulty with their balance. With persistence and discipline, distractibility will lessen and new emergent properties of awareness will develop. Meditation is not a skill to master and move on from but a practice to relish and maintain relationship with and evolve with throughout one's life. As with any skill it takes work to develop and work to maintain, so practice, practice, practice.

As one continues to concentrate and attend to the moment, focus becomes a subtle art, and moments of ultimate balance and supreme stillness arise. The experience of a constant subtle vibration of energy exists everywhere at once. This makes balance elusive and ever changing, and the path to seeking it is dynamic and alive, shifting in relationship to our experience and leading us to ever-emerging phenomena.

With daily practice we find the fulcrum of balance, like that of a seesaw when two children on either end participate in the interplay of a dynamic movement between the two sides. It is a living process, a volley between extremes, until our awareness becomes so refined that a struggle is no longer necessary. Although vast stillness is not typically a part of most people's normal daily perceptions, the ebb and flow of awareness of this depth of stillness is present.

As we balance on the tightrope of attention during meditation, a one-pointed focus comes in and out of our experience. From the finite perspective of one-pointed focus we can develop a multifocal and, ultimately, infinitely refined focus that deepens into profound stillness. Insight comes from the wellspring of stillness and can lead us to the rich place of infinite awareness. But it's here one moment, gone the next. We pay attention to breath as it flows in and out of our lungs, our thoughts, and our feelings and passes through the spotlight of our mind in a flash. Inhale—an emotion, exhale—another moment gone. This is meditation practice. The beginning steps to becoming still become a lived experience, and we can sense the possibilities ahead. A breathless state of grace awakens us. Initially these insights are fleeting, but with time they can become more established and profound.

The most profound change we can make is to move toward balance: finding pleasure in routine and in daily tasks. We can get up at the same time each and every day, eat a simple, whole-foods diet, speak in calm and humble truths, and spend time in the natural world. As we surrender to the natural order, patterns of awareness develop, the body finds healing, and the mind grows calmer. The human being becomes attuned to a cosmic alignment and life is more joyful.

## THE GIFT OF PATANJALI'S YOGA SUTRAS: AN EIGHTFOLD PATH

The Yoga Sutras of Patanjali is considered to be the oldest systematic written account of the integrated discipline and practice of yoga.

# Patanjali's (octave) Yoga Sutras

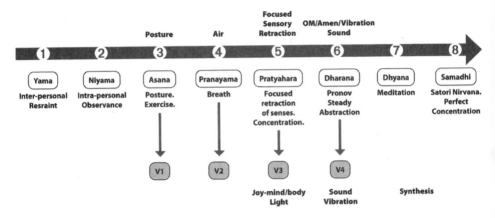

Figure 4.2. Patanjali's eightfold path.

Although thought to be written several thousand years ago, it didn't become well known until the 1900s, when its value was rediscovered. The work structures the practice of yoga into an eight-step process (see figure 4.2) that addresses many of the struggles we face every day in current society. It is also considered an outline for a vibrant life.

The gift of Patanjali's eightfold path is that it reaches all humans across time and space, culture and race, suffering and survival to offer simple guidance toward Self-Realization. The first two limbs, *yama* and *niyama,* highlight traits worth developing and lay a groundwork for moral conduct. Note that limbs 3 through 6—asana, pranayama, *pratyahara,* and *dharana,* respectively—correspond to the four stages of Kriya yoga given in the Cycle of Synthesis as V1 to V4, and limbs 7 (*dhyana*) and 8 (*samadhi*) correspond to meditation and Self-Realization, or perfect concentration, respectively, all of which were discussed in chapter 4.

The self-regulating behaviors of yama and niyama help us to create the balance we discussed earlier in this chapter. The yamas are interpersonal restraints, and the niyamas are intrapersonal observances. In other words, they are the dos and don'ts for a contented life and are not unlike the Ten

Commandments or Buddha's eightfold path. The yamas and niyamas are perhaps relatively obvious ways to live a life of correct action, yet it seems to be a tall task for humanity to attain this goal collectively. Therefore, we all must make a greater effort individually to seek to neutralize negative behaviors in our own lives and help others to do the same. Ganesh Baba found that the practice of Kriya yoga brought out the interpersonal restraints and intrapersonal observances in an individual automatically.

The five interpersonal yamas include the following:

1. Nonviolence (*ahimsa*)—Not harming other living creatures with words or actions and cultivating a feeling of benevolence in oneself is the first goal.
2. Truthfulness (*satya*)—Speaking truth and holding truth in one's mind is essential to living in alignment. Progressive practice of Kriya yoga makes it next to impossible to be untrue in speech or thought.
3. Nonstealing/Trustworthiness (*asteya*)—Being trustworthy and not stealing from others is important for creating a world where others may rely on you to have their best interest at heart.
4. Nonexcess (*brahmacharya*)—Using mental and physical self-restraint when thinking, talking, attempting to take action, and taking action. It is also to have correct thoughts regarding sexuality in relation to spiritual health (see the box on page 54).
5. Nonattachment or nonpossessiveness (*aparigraha*)—Having only that which is needed without hoarding or being greedy. Nonattachment does not mean a lack of love, respect, or caring. It refers to a mild mind that is adaptable and capable of supporting self and others in unconditional peace.

The five intrapersonal niyamas are as follows:

1. Self-discipline (*tapas*)—Practicing perseverance like that in persistent meditation. Without regular practice and the fortitude to follow through, few results will be made manifest.

2. Self-observation, introspection and study of scripture (*svadhyaya*)—
Engaging in a contemplative practice that requires ongoing self-
analysis and some exposure to sacred texts. Scriptures have truths
that resonate with people differently and participating or reading
scriptures can awaken new perspectives within oneself and lead
one's heart to progress along the path.

3. Remembering Nature/Spirit (*isvarapranidhana*)—Having cognitive
awareness of the Absolute, or Divine. Rejoicing in Mother Nature.

4. Mental and physical cleanliness (*sauca*): Taking care of one's body-
mind-spirit and treating it as a temple for the expression of God.

5. Contentment (*santosa*)—Feeling that what you have is enough,
regarding all things. It is not abandonment but extreme acceptance
with action and intention whether it be inner or outer.

. . . . . . . . . . . . . . . . . . . . . . . . . . . . . . . . . . . . . . . . . . . .

### Further Note on Brahmacharya and Celibacy

Sexuality and spiritual practice can often become confusing as
there is very little deep understanding regarding the interactions
of innate biological sexual libido, psychological dynamics, trauma,
lust, love, compassion, power, loneliness, safety, and attachments/
bonding. This list only scratches the surface of the complicated
dynamics involved in intimate sexual activity with another living
and breathing being. In spiritual practices these issues are further
confused due to the long-standing practice of celibacy in many religious and spiritual traditions. It is certainly clear that removing the
allure of sexuality from a certain environment allows for concentration and focus on other things such as spiritual practice. Our
libido is an incredibly strong, divine, creative drive of Nature, as it
is throughout the animal kingdom, and none of us would be here
without it. In fact, our lives depend on sexuality, but our evolution
and survival depend on spirituality.

Celibacy or staying away from environments where sexual
relationships are expected or encouraged can be helpful for a
young aspiring individual who is trying to find their footing in the

world of the contemplative sciences. Being able to shift the normal physiological drive for sexual intimacy to compassion and spiritual awareness can be helpful for a period of time, although that is not to say that celibacy is a requirement for spiritual transcendence. Sexuality in itself does not lead to enlightenment although spiritual awakening can lead to more enlightened sexuality. It is with this in mind that one can come to an understanding that no path is the same and all paths have risks.

. . . . . . . . . . . . . . . . . . . . . . . . . . . . . . . . . . . . . . . . . . . . . . . . . .

We would do well to understand that contentment does not come in the form of material things but rather through giving to others, accepting others, remaining optimistic in life, and making a connection to higher Self. The yamas and niyamas, the Upanishads, the Bhagavad Gita, and the Brahma Sutras provide a foundation for what is often referred to as Vedanta. They make philosophical suggestions and add a devotional aspect to the niyamas such as a belief in an energy and intelligence beyond us. These writings make up the central core of a spiritual path and include forgiveness, fortitude, compassion, sincerity, and a measured diet. Studying scripture is included, as well as having remorse and acceptance of one's past actions, maintaining modesty and humility, reflecting deeply on thought, and engaging in mantra. The Indian scriptures, Buddha's Four Noble Truths, middle way, and eight-fold path, the Ten Commandments, and others provide the building blocks of balance for inter- and intrapersonal action, thought, speech, and behavior. With Kriya yoga it is expected that the yamas and niyamas will develop on their own and rather quickly if one is engaged in consistent practice.

# PART II

## PRACTICING KRIYA YOGA

# 5

# Spiritualization, the Cycle of Synthesis, and the Four Vs of Kriya

*To enjoy synchronicity in one's life journey is a blessing.*

We are at a time in history where the speed of transmission is an important aspect of spiritualization, which again is the process of activating our physiology toward further human evolution. This may sound like an oxymoron but consider the level of continual distractions we are faced with daily: the stress of employment circumstances, the high cost of living, and the expanding fear-based mentality thriving on the planet. With the advent of cultural exchange through travel, media, and technology, it seems that time has increased its velocity but left us in its wake, and our collective level of consciousness is suffering.

This has led to a rather bleak existence with an ever-increasing pursuit of material comforts, feelings of isolation, and illusions of separation. This is partly because we doubt our own experience in general and our experience of the Divine in particular. If we seek pleasures that are transient in their ability to sustain happiness, we engage in a tireless effort to seek satisfaction at the expense of all else. That leaves us with emptiness and obsession, but it can also open a door to spiritualization and the ways we can bring it about. As mentioned in previous chapters, meditation and breath are two avenues with which to explore our deeper desires as humans for a wisdom that transcends our base physical desires. Once we are able to touch that with our whole being, we are clearly on the path of truth and it is hard to turn around. And the compass that will lead us to this clarity is prana.

Prana, life force, is the energy that enables us to find a convergence between biological science and Spirit and provides an interface between our gross body and our spiritual body. If there is one particular facet of Kriya yoga that is essential, it is finding the prana in our own breath. This is the first phase in cultivating appreciation for prana, the life-force energy of Mother Nature that lives within us. By focusing within the physical body, our breath becomes the channel to the endless central reservoir of this energy. It is through breath-focused exercises, concentration, and immersion that we can access and quiet the mind: stillness of breath equals stillness of mind. It is this juncture between body and mind, prana and science that can help to illustrate the concept of spiritualization, a model to represent the human experience.

## A DETAILED LOOK AT THE CYCLE OF SYNTHESIS

To help us understand the human experience and gain access to spiritualization, Ganesh Baba created a system with four energetic fields that represent an extrapolation of the electromagnetic spectrum beyond the space-time continuum, which is beyond the speed of light. This system, which he called the Cycle of Synthesis (see figure 5.1 on page 60), provides a model that integrates theory, technique, philosophy, and science with a quantum perspective. I have been able to enjoy this model of the human experience for the last forty years and it continues to provide insights for me in personal, professional, and spiritual areas of my life.

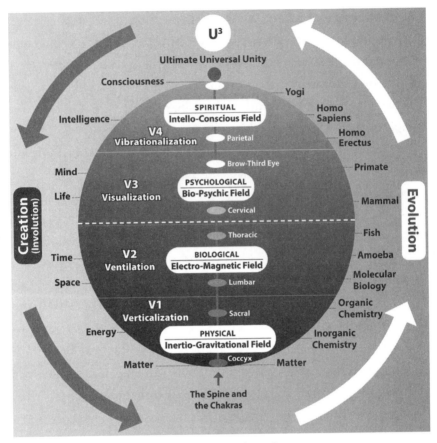

Figure 5.1. Cycle of Synthesis.

In Kriya yoga, as taught by Ganesh Baba, the Cycle of Synthesis is a two-dimensional model on which to hang a description of an eight-dimensional lived experience. It is an attempt to create a working example that describes what we know to have infinite dimensional potential. This framework is a way to help categorize information in a meaningful cohesive fashion so that our mind can better grasp the relationships of these aspects of our experience. The four fields of the Cycle of Synthesis combined with the concepts of quantum physics offer us a mandala, or a circular model of the cosmos, to describe creation and evolution through a synthesis of the Vedanta, yoga, tantra (see box on page 61), and modern science.

These four fields are named the inertio-gravitational, electro-magnetic, bio-psychic and intello-conscious and represent respectively the physical, physiological, psychological, and spiritual aspects of human experience. These fields are modeled after the electromagnetic spectrum, which includes light, electricity, and the wireless communication we use in our daily lives. As in the electromagnetic field, the flow of the electron is the current (electricity) that manifests the magnetic field around it. Turn off the current and the field is gone. On the other hand, movement of a magnet or a magnetic field can also cause an electrical current. This idea of the relationship between current and field is repeated in the other three fields as an extrapolation of the basic idea of energy. An example we have already spoken about is the current of life producing the field of the mind. The electromagnetic spectrum is most easily recognized by observing the visual spectrum of light and colors, which include red, orange, yellow, green, blue, indigo, and violet.

· · · · · · · · · · · · · · · · · · · · · · · · · · · · · · · · · · · · · · · · · · · · ·

## Tantra

Tantra as it relates to Kriya yoga is a set of energetic practices that have been largely misunderstood as sexual in nature. Tantra literature often refers to the masculine and feminine principles in speaking about spirituality and transcendence. Many words in the literature have meanings dramatically different from those that appear on the surface. In general, the references are to the creative aspect of Nature, the feminine principle, and the masculine aspect of the Spirit, experienced as awareness. Tantra, like yoga, is about union; not a physical sensual union, but the union of yin and yang, masculine and feminine, positive and negative, Spirit and Nature, or in Indian philosophy, Shiva and Shakti that occurs in states of stillness when one's inhalation intertwines with the exhalation in a moment of stillness, sometimes referred to as breathlessness or the merging of prana and aprana. This is the philosophy and practice of tantra. It is an internal practice of one's relationship with Mother Nature in her grandest most universal form. It is not focused on touch or sexual intimacy with another human being. Tantra is all about the experience of the Divine and is described in the Indian scriptures as kundalini, Self-Realization, God realization, and samadhi, among others. Kriya yoga as taught by Ganesh Baba is the essence of tantra and yoga combined.

. . . . . . . . . . . . . . . . . . . . . . . . . . . . . . . . . . . . . . . . . . . . . . .

The left side of the Cycle of Synthesis depicts creation—Cosmic Consciousness coming into matter—while the right side represents the evolution of matter returning to Cosmic Consciousness by way of development through human life. The creation side of the cycle has eight categories that attempt to describe and categorize the human experience. They reflect the ideas of Immanuel Kant, who spoke about a priori knowledge or categories of knowledge that exist independent of experience. This represents the domains of human existence that do not require our awareness of them in order to exist. At the same time, does anything exist without awareness? The basic idea is that without awareness these are simply the *potential* categories of human experience and with awareness they manifest in consciousness as our *actual* human experience. These "Kantian" categories, as named by Ganesh Baba are matter, energy, space, time, life, mind, intelligence, and consciousness.

In the Cycle of Synthesis the four lower categories—matter, energy, space, and time—which make up the inertio-gravitational and electro-magnetic fields and represent the space-time continuum as understood by our current scientific models. As we move up the cycle we come to the four upper categories—life, mind, intelligence, and consciousness—which make up the bio-psychic and intello-conscious fields and are energies that we currently cannot measure directly with our state of technology. For although we can measure the by-products of life with electronic instruments such as EEGs and ECGs or use our own senses to feel someone's heart rate or watch someone breathe, we cannot identify an individual's specific thoughts or measure an emotion in any objective sense. We can measure what life does, but not where it comes from or where it goes. We cannot measure how many breaths or how much life force remains in anyone's lifetime with any of our current meters. These upper two energetic fields are beyond what is considered part of the four-dimensional space-time continuum from the measurement standpoint. Nonetheless we do not deny that our life force is real even though we cannot measure it directly. The cycle is also separated into a top and bottom half by a dashed line that represents the linear interface of time, with which we measure our life. This is the interface where the four-dimensional space-time continuum interfaces with energetic fields that are beyond time. This is the energetic area that we currently can only measure with our human biopsychic instrument, our felt experience.

The evolution side of the Cycle of Synthesis demonstrates movement going upward from the most basic elements of matter to inorganic and organic molecules and then moving into life and along the path of evolution as described by Darwin. On the left side of the cycle we see the eight Kantian categories, which by themselves or in some combination represent the varieties of the human experience. This humancentric idea suggests that we are the pinnacle of biological evolution while yogic philosophy proposes that Darwinian biological evolution is merely the initial frontier for human evolution, which is now posed to move into higher states of conscious evolution by the practices of Kriya and similar techniques.

In this model the fields of energy are extrapolated from the well-understood concepts of the electromagnetic spectrum (see figure 5.2 on page 64). The photon is the discreet packet of electromagnetic energy. It travels at the speed of light and propagates its energy with the properties of both a particle and wave. The theory as proposed in the Cycle of Synthesis is that the other three fields have corresponding quanta, or packets of energy. The inertio-gravitational field theoretical quanta is referred to as a graviton, the bio-psychic field has the bion, and the intello-conscious field has the assigned name of consion.

The figure shows that visual light is only a small fraction of the overall electromagnetic spectrum and depicts the behavior changes

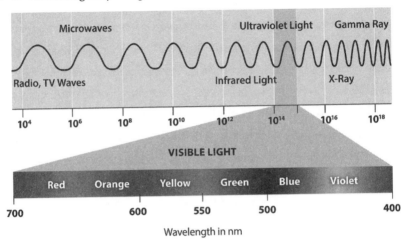

Figure 5.2. Electromagnetic spectrum.

relative to frequency and wavelength, i.e., the frequency increases as the wavelength decreases, thus changing the behavior of the energy from a radio wave, to visible light, to X-rays.

This pattern theoretically continues with the shift in energy and velocity from one field to the next. The two lowest fields—inertio-gravitational and electro-magnetic—are the most matter-infused, while the higher bio-psychic and intello-conscious fields are energetic without physical properties. The photon, the quanta of energy in the electromagnetic field moves at the speed of light. As we move higher up in the fields to the bio-psychic and intello-conscious fields we see an increase in the frequency, the energy of the specific quanta, and the speed of motion in each successive energy field. In this model, this culminates (or actually originates) in the intello-conscious field with the consion. The consion is described as having infinite velocity, meaning that it is present at every point in space at every moment, therefore transcending both time and space. An attempt at a definition of God from the standpoint of modern physics. The energies in these fields intermingle and influence each other. The intello-conscious field permeates all others with equal intensity, while the inertio-gravitational field has the least effect on the upper fields. This model serves to provide some structure for ideas that generally defied language as a means to describe them.

In the terms of modern physics these higher field energies are ethereal, yet are very real and experienced by many. The breath exercises presented in Kriya yoga teach us how to feel into and modulate these energy fields by presenting various ways of changing our awareness until it opens up into the intello-conscious field, guiding us to the direct experience of the Absolute, or U3. The chakras are depicted in the cycle as the straight vertical line that separates the right and left sides and represents our central nervous system. In fact, each of the four main practices in Kriya, V1 through V4, correspond with a particular field and thus function as a way to integrate these aspects of our being as we practice Kriya and move toward deeper states of meditation. This experience leaves long-lasting changes in our neuronal networks as well as in the other energy fields, contributing to a greater sense of equanimity in life. A feeling of deep pervasive relaxation and embodied joy spills into the whole body and mind. With time one learns to modulate these energies within a moment's notice and is able to share altruistic love, intuition, and synchronicity (see box below) in ways that were previously experienced in fleeting moments but can now be utilized as easily as spoken language. In fact, these communications are outside of language and outside of our normal space-time continuum.

Notice that the diagram in figure 5.1 on page 60 shows that the Cycle of Synthesis itself is set on the field of the U3, the background from which the first breath arises and the undifferentiated ground of nonduality. The Cycle of Synthesis, then, is representing a model of creation from that instant that is just behind the big bang; the moment when the dance of the first vibration began to form the ultimate stillness of U3.

. . . . . . . . . . . . . . . . . . . . . . . . . . . . . . . . . . . . . . . . . . . . .

### Kriya Yoga and Synchronicity

One fringe benefit of practicing Kriya yoga is often a marked increase in synchronicity, an increase of resonance that is outside our normal waking consciousness. *Synchronicity* is a term first used by Carl Jung and described in his book on the topic as "an acausal

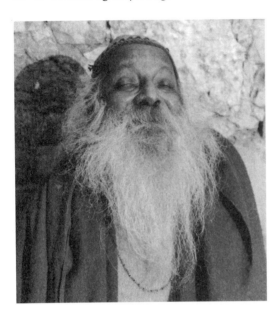

Figure 5.3. Ganesh Baba, touching the Infinite. (Photo by Michelle Cruzel.)

connecting principle." It is a term used to describe meaningful co-occurrences that do not have a causal link. *The Merriam-Webster Dictionary* describes synchronicity as "the coincidental occurrence of events that seem related but are not explained by the conventional mechanisms of causality." In other words, some events meaningfully coincide at a particular moment but without any traditional linear connection prior to that synchronistic moment. Other words used to describe a similar phenomenon are *coincidence, grace, resonance,* and *luck.* Those terms vary considerably in their underlying meaning and have more to do with the individual assigning the word to the phenomenon than the phenomenon itself.

It is my experience that through the practice of Kriya yoga, synchronicity increases in life exponentially in relation to one's practice. Although the Absolute is beyond time and space, our bodies and minds are still influenced by the four dimensions of the space-time continuum. By practicing Kriya yoga we can transcend those limitations while at the same time staying grounded within this space-time continuum for everyday matters such as sustenance, security, shelter, and sex/reproduction. That said, the practice of Kriya yoga decreases our desires and attachments for all four of these categories. Sustenance becomes just that, as the Kriya yogi is no longer looking for icing on the cake. Security, although a concern for others, is less a concern for Kriya yogis as they have already tasted the ultimate security of the Divine. Of course, shelter is pleasant but the barest accommodations are sufficient.

With regard to sexuality, the physical orgasm loses much of its attraction as the orgasmic qualities of the Divine allow for extended periods of time to be spent in the orgasmic moment of bliss as opposed to a fleeting moment during sexual activity. As one continues to practice these techniques, energies in the body shift, and synchronicity begins to interweave with the Kriya yogi in a more familiar fashion, lightening the load and enlightening the path. Although synchronicity is occurring outside of space and time, it is connected to the person who is in space and time, and it is this interaction of the space-time continuum and beyond that synchronicity demonstrates to us so beautifully.

Synchronicity can be an important factor in moving forward along the path to the Divine and should not be ignored when it presents itself. It is grace in motion, and no amount of energetic practice can bring back a lost moment of grace. In fact, the more you can maintain mindful heartfelt awareness throughout the day, the better your attunement will be for attracting synchronicity into your life. Be present, as to not be present is to not be there at all.

Welcome to Kriya yoga.

. . . . . . . . . . . . . . . . . . . . . . . . . . . . . . . . . . . . . . . . . . . . . .

## KRIYA YOGA AND SPIRITUALIZATION

There are four initial exercise stages on the Kriya yoga path to spiritualization (see figure 5.4 on page 68): verticalization (V1), ventilation (V2), visualization (V3), and vibrationalization (V4). Each exercise corresponds to one of the four fields previously referred to in the Cycle of Synthesis. V1 refers to posture and corresponds to the inertiogravitational field, which relates to our physical body. V2 relates to the breath, and it comes from the Indian practice of pranayama (yogic breath exercises) and involves our biology. V3 refers to the inner light, our mind's eye, and engages our mind. V4 refers to the use of a sound, mantra, or a short phrase to help steady language-based thoughts while at the same time providing a rhythmic sound pattern to help resonate with what is described as "the unstruck sound," Om (Aum) or "The Word." To work with your mind, you'll have to be patient; you'll have to cultivate a collaborative working relationship with yourself and your posture and your breath, which ultimately controls the mind.

These exercises when combined contribute to a solid stable physical base that is calmed by regular, reposed, rhythmic respiration and internal visual focus and language centers that are quieted by concentrating on the third eye and repetitive sound/vibration. This leads to increasing stillness with internal focus and with time develops a new pattern of interaction between aspects of environment within our central nervous system that allows meditation, a new emergent property for which the brain is already wired, to blossom and come to life.

## Verticalization (V1)

Posture is the first and most important step in Kriya yoga because physical structure is where the practice begins. The spine must be stable,

### Kriya Yoga
**The Basics – The Work**

| V1 | Verticalization | Posture |
|----|-----------------|---------|
| V2 | Ventilation | Breath |
| V3 | Visualization | Third Eye |
| V4 | Vibrationalization | Mantra |
| | **Meditation** | |

Maintain your own religion or belief system.

Figure 5.4. Four Kriya Yoga practices. In previous writings about Ganesh Baba's Kriya yoga these four practices are referred to as the 4 Ps: posture, pranayama, pratyahara, and pronov (pranava). In keeping with the goal of making this an English language publication, the four Ps are now the four Vs: verticalization, ventilation, visualization, and vibrationalization.

supportive, supple, and erect to provide for clear reception and optimal respiration. Think of your spine, or central canal, as an antenna with which to tune in to the body and its energy fields. From the crown to the coccyx, it brings light and life into the body. Ideally, our spine is always maintained in its anatomically correct position as a column and not hunched over like an arch. Take a look at figure 5.5 below and spend a few minutes breathing into this idea.

## Ventilation (V2)

Breath is the energy behind Kriya yoga meditation. As the breath goes so goes the mind. The breath helps to quiet the mind and allows meditation to spring forth. We work on posture in V1 to allow for full respiration in V2 so that our mind can calm and focus internally. Normal respiration can only occur with an anatomically correct posture. In figure 5.6 on page 70 you can see that as the diaphragm contracts (see the box on page 71 for more details on the diaphragm), it creates a vacuum in the thoracic cavity that is filled as the air comes in. As this is occurring the chest expands and the ribs move up and out (assisted by accessory muscles) to increase the volume in the chest cavity so it can hold more air. On exhalation all these muscles relax and the air is easily exhaled. Many individuals, even when doing breathing exercises, allow the chest to collapse on

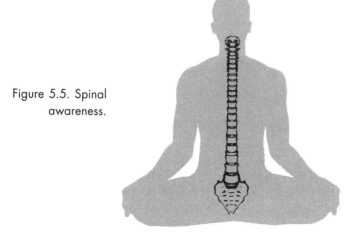

Figure 5.5. Spinal awareness.

exhalation. In Kriya yoga, however, the goal on exhalation is to maintain an erect spine with a chest that is still relatively expanded, as it was when filled with air, and the chest certainly does not collapse.

It is ultimately the so-called breathless state that corresponds to deeper states of meditation. When breath fills the lungs with air, oxygen is carried with it, providing life to every cell. And each cell participates in its own active cellular version of respiration, which occurs at all times. The goal is to have regular, reposed, rhythmic respiration that, with time, becomes your regular pattern of breathing. Practice bringing breath into the body slowly and sending energy intentionally to various areas of the body. Explore your breath. As the incoming breath expands your chest, taste it, feel it, touch it inside, hold it, embrace it, and release it once again for the next cycle. Learn to savor each inhalation; it is a friend, a good friend who always comes back around for more. With time and practice of the 4 Vs the breath can spontaneously become so subtle that one can appear breathless. This subtle yet dynamic breath, which usually accompanies deep states of meditation, is sometimes referred to as Kriya breath or Kriya pranayama.

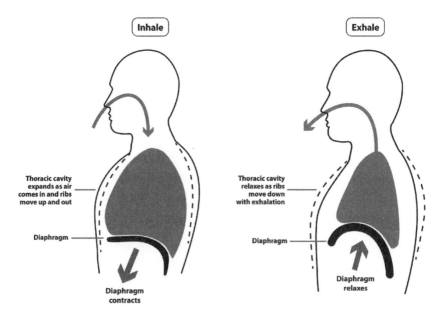

Figure 5.6. Normal respiration.

## The Diaphragm's Role in Respiration

The actions that contribute to our ability to inhale and exhale are complex and highly integrated. The reflex to breathe is one of our deepest drives and overcomes many obstacles in both physical illness and psychological distress and allows us to keep functioning or at least stay alive. Even when the system has enough oxygen to function any significant distress in the system can and does have a negative impact on our autonomic nervous system and can lead to a mismatch between the parasympathetic nervous system and the sympathetic nervous system causing anxiety, distress, unease, fear, and anger. Respiratory illness such as asthma, heart failure, and COPD lead to the stress of not being able to catch your breath and put strain on all the muscles involved in taking a breath.

This is the reason that posture is important for proper respiration, which, again, is the foundation of Kriya meditation. The diaphragm, intercostal muscles, shoulder girdle, paraspinal muscles, scalene muscles, rhomboid muscles, and even the neck muscles are all involved with our ability to take in a breath and let it out. The diaphragm is one of the largest muscles of the body. It is shaped like a dome or an open umbrella and separates the thorax from the abdomen. It has a central tendon and touches the thorax and aspects of the ribs and lumbar vertebrae. It also attaches to the fascia that cover organs of the thorax including the pericardium, which covers the heart and the pleura, which cover the lungs. The diaphragm allows the esophagus, aorta, and vena cava to pass through it, going from the thorax to the abdominal cavity.

Diaphragm dysfunction can negatively affect posture, attention, energy level, mood, gastrointestinal function, breath, and heart rate and can cause anxiety, anger, back pain, and headaches. Physical and psychological trauma can negatively affect the diaphragm and its function. Many people have experienced states in dreams or life-threatening situations when the ability to talk or scream seems to vanish. Being punched in the solar plexus also renders someone breathless and unable to speak. These are examples of how the diaphragm can get frozen with a body memory that cannot readily be expressed in words, as the expression of language was impaired at the time of the trauma. It is these experiences that can be helped with somatic psychotherapies, auricular acupuncture-assisted psychotherapy, and pranayama, as well as bodywork such as cranial osteopathy that assists in releasing the diaphragm.

A basic grasp of the diaphragm's anatomy is helpful in understanding how it affects respiration. As you can see in figure 5.7, the diaphragm even attaches to the lumbar vertebrae. The significance of this is that full respiration cannot occur with a low back that is not in its anatomically correct position, as it would put strain on the diaphragm and limit its movement. Once again, we arrive back to the point of maintaining an anatomically correct spinal position for optimal function.

### Visualization (V3)

Fine-tuning inner vision makes the first glimpse of unity possible. This typically entails focusing one's attention on the area between the eyebrows, a point that goes by a few different names, including the *ajna* chakra, gyral center, *kutasha,* mind's eye, inner sky, and third eye. In the beginning, practice becoming more aware of the third eye's energy.

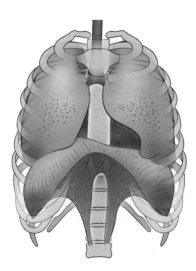

Figure 5.7. Diaphragm.

As you focus there you will begin to notice that your inner field of vision can be adjusted from pinpointed precision to open and broad, an inner peripheral vision if you will. It is best to use attention and let the eyes do as they will at first. The problem with starting with actually moving your eyes to look at the third eye (Shambhavi mudra) is the inherent shakiness of the eyeball in such a position. This ends up being a distraction as stillness is important. It is fine to experiment and see for yourself. With time one typically uses both techniques at different times to aid the meditative process or explore other effects. Starting with attention first will likely be easier and more productive. This is an example of micromodulation, which we talk about later on. Once you have practiced posture and breath for a while, the third eye often comes into focus with little effort. In time one's attention is almost magnetically pulled to it, and it appears clear as day. This often corresponds to a sense of pleasure and deep relaxation. During this practice keep your eyebrows slightly raised, yet still relaxed. One can even find that the corners of your mouth will turn upward in an open expression of friendly invitation. This is a very important aspect of the Kriya yoga practice. It is an entry point to Infinity.

### Vibrationalization (V4)

All of life is intelligent and carries a unique vibrational footprint. During this step it is beneficial to practice a sound or mantra such as *Om*, or *Aum*, and connect to the universal sound called pronov. Try to vocalize *Om* (*Aum*) with four syllables—aaah, oooh, mmm—or just make a humming sound. Note that the fourth syllable is the silence, the absence of any sound that occurs both before and after Om.

Of course, if other variations of mantra like *amen* resonate better with you, practice those. Other sounds—short prayerful phrases,* as well as musical scales or humming—can also be used as an auditory focus, and some individuals experience a spontaneous phrase or

---

*Examples of other sacred syllables include: *omen, hum, ameen, satnam,* and *ram* among others.

sound that can be used as well. There is no need for a complicated mantra. Om is more than sufficient. What is important is flow and cadence. Find something that you resonate with. With time, any repetitive sound will take on a vibrational energy of its own, fine-tuning your meditative experience and bringing it additional focus and power.

Just as one can visualize something and keep it in the mind's eye, one can also hear something and keep it in the mind's ear. This is what V4 is ultimately about. With time one can hear the inner vibration, the pronov, as it is within as much as it is without. One way to experience this is with a gong, tuning fork, cymbal, or metal meditation singing bowl such as those often seen in meditation centers. Such a bell is often rung to signal the beginning or end of meditation, and the sound of the bell reverberates throughout the entire environment and into the being of those present. Hearing a church bell reverberate over the land has a similar effect. Listen closely to the sound, as it fades from your ears you'll continue to hear it in your mind's ear. This is the beginning of training one's ability to tune in to the primordial vibration—the hum of the cosmos, the eternal Om, the unstruck sound. Cover both your ears. What do you hear?

### The Four Vs and Meditation

The synchronization of these four exercises, V1, V2, V3, and V4, result in the next stage, which is meditation itself. Meditation is an emergent property that occurs when these four exercises become second nature and begin to support one another in an effortless flow. Short periods of time spent engaged in these tasks will be sufficient in the early stages. Over time the practitioner will build stamina and be able to maintain longer periods of contemplation. As one is more able to resonate with breath and spirit, building connection with the directable energy of prana, toning the lungs, and aligning the body, deeper meditative states will occur, and synchronicities will happen with increasing regularity.

## HUMANITY AND THE APTITUDE FOR SPIRITUALIZATION

The Cycle of Synthesis is a conceptual model that describes the land-scape of experience, but it is not to be understood as the experience itself. The philosophy put forth in the Cycle of Synthesis is an attempt to provide a framework for meaningful interactions with and the results from a Kriya yoga breathwork practice. It also serves as a reference point to help ground perspective in the cognitive, meditation-based language, so our minds may better compile and integrate psychospiritual information. Meditation is simply a process of learning to manage power and energy in a focused way within our physical, biological, psychological, and spiritual selves and then following the path that opens before us.

Of course, Kriya yoga is not alone in proposing that humans move forward to develop an aptitude for spiritualization in this way. Historically, this path has been pursued by those seeking some form of enlightenment. It is now more possible than ever to learn methods and techniques for attaining peace in one's life. Rigidity in one or another type of yoga, such as karma, bhakti, jnana, or hatha, is unnecessary and counterproductive, as all paths in yoga lead to a similar place. Such a deeply evolved system as yoga has a combination for everyone.

The Indian spiritual traditions are an integrated web of practices each of which resonates with different individuals, making the journey easier, quicker, and more enjoyable. Once one has success in a particular self-regulatory technique, one may receive great insight in the ability to enter and modulate other such techniques. The spiritual experience is not unique to an individual or culture and although the paths or belief systems may differ, the deep physiological changes and the ability to experience the U3 is ubiquitous among all spiritual pursuits. Kriya is available to all and in fact may play a role in helping one find which path they resonate with most. These practices are nonsectarian while at the same time being the underlying essence of all religion. All humans can access these fields of experience just as we all learn to walk and talk.

# 6

# Spine Bolt Upright

## Posture as a Fast-Track to the Infinite

*Posture, posture, posture.*

So far we have considered the genius of Ganesh Baba, the roots and foundation of Kriya yoga and its connection to the many other yoga traditions, introduced the four basic practices of Kriya, the gifts of Buddha and Patanjali, and the paths one might follow to find one's own ideal spiritual practice. We have also discussed the Cycle of Synthesis, which attempts to integrate the brilliant wisdom of Darwin and Kant with the Vedas and modern science. Hopefully these topics have opened the door to a new perspective on the depth of yoga.

None of what has been shared is secret or hidden intentionally. This information on Kriya yoga is offered openly to any person who seeks it. This particular form, as passed on through Ganesh Baba, weaves together these many different schools of thought to create a direct and efficient practice that is both teachable and attainable by the motivated student. If there is anything that bridges these concepts with seamless integrity, it is doing the work of pranayama, or breath exercises, on a sound postural structure.

Most meditation trainings and much of the literature make only a passing reference to posture. Some teachers will stress the importance of posture, but most trainings and writings have little focus on the spine other than a passing mention to sit up straight. However, as mentioned earlier, nearly every statue of Buddha, Shiva, Ganesh, and others shows an upright posture that is almost divine in perfection (see figure 6.1).

One can spend hours sitting in meditation, but if it's done with a hunched posture rather than a fully erect spine, then one cannot engage the full capacity of breath. And if one cannot breathe properly, how then can one expect to engage the entirety of what it means to be human, much less explore the cosmos?

In Kriya training, it is the foundation of a strong, straight, and flexible spine that guarantees that a practitioner will experience moments of great joy and compassion and deep insights. And these higher states of consciousness are not just for mystics; they can be achieved with a deep commitment to a Kriya yoga practice that brings one into alignment with oneself.

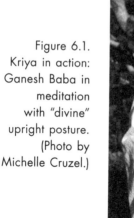
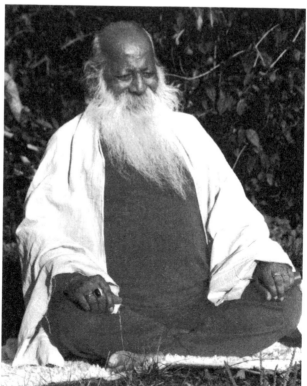

Figure 6.1.
Kriya in action:
Ganesh Baba in
meditation
with "divine"
upright posture.
(Photo by
Michelle Cruzel.)

We are energetic beings—part physical, part biological, part mind, and part spirit. We are animated by the energy of Nature and Spirit through a body and form, and it is our honor and responsibility to care for this being and use it to integrate the four areas of posture, breath, mind, and spirit (V1–V4) so that we can experience resonance, altruistic love, and universal unity, or as Yogananda expressed it:

> The spine and the brain are the altars of God. That's where the electricity of God flows down into the nervous system and into the world. And the searchlights of your senses are turned outwards. But when you reverse the searchlights, through Kriya yoga, and will be concentrated in the spine, you will behold the Maker.
>
> That's what Self-Realization teaches: The technique of meditation, recharging the body battery with cosmic energy—for it is not a creed or dogma, but a science of the soul and spirit. How the soul descended from the Cosmic Consciousness into the earth and the body and the senses, is the purpose of this work.[1]

## SPINAL AWARENESS

Figure 6.2 shows three examples of proper meditation posture. Notice that even the statue of Buddha is showing the spine as a column and not an arch.

Verticalization (V1), or posture, is the first and most important step in the practice of Kriya yoga. The spine must be stable, supportive, supple, and erect to provide for clear reception (see figure 6.3 on page 80). The vertebrae make up a carefully crafted column of individual building blocks. When they are balanced one on top of the other, they hold our weight in an effortless fashion. In addition, a properly aligned posture allows for the muscles and bones of respiration to do their job without stress or stain. This is the secret to stilling the mind.

In the center of the spinal cord, which is contained within the bony

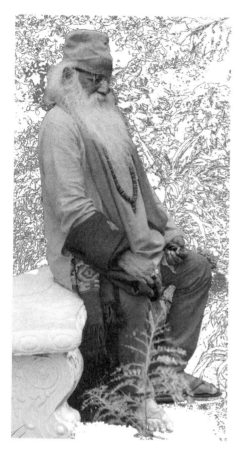

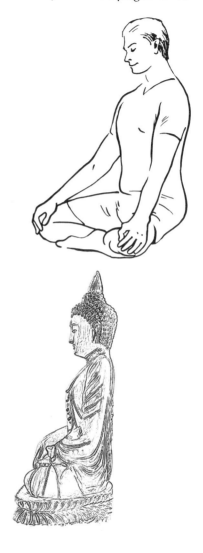

Figure 6.2. Three examples of proper meditation posture. Ganesh Baba is shown in meditation at Self-Realization's Mount Washington in Los Angeles, California in the early 1980s. (Photo of Ganesh Baba by Keith Lowenstein.)

structure of the spine, is a small canal the width of a pin called the central canal (see figure 6.4 on page 81). Some of our cerebrospinal fluid flows through this canal, and it is easy to see that any significant distortion of the spinal column could impede the flow of this most precious bodily fluid. This inner canal of the spinal cord, also considered the *sushumna,* has great significance in the practice of yogic meditation. It is considered the center of one's antennae, the area where the

Figure 6.3. The brain and spinal cord make up the central nervous system, as pictured here. In addition to performing its traditional physiological function, you can think of the brain with spinal cord as being your antennae to the subtle energies of human experence.

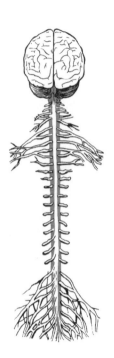

spiritual energy known as kundalini* appears to travel in the spine and beyond. Currently there is no Western scientific measurement of this energy, although it has proven to be reproducible across the globe over thousands of years by the practitioners of the contemplative arts.

## THE ANATOMY OF PROPER POSTURE

Proper posture is of the utmost importance in facilitating the process of meditation, just as it is in playing golf, dancing, singing, or riding a bicycle. One's posture in Kriya yoga provides the stability of a solid yet supple and alive structural support on which the biological, psycho-

---

*Kundalini is a term used to describe a potential energetic pattern that can become kinetic or active spontaneously or during specific meditation techniques and is associated with Self-Realization. It is described as traveling through the sushumna, an energy pathway with the closest anatomical correlate being the central canal of the spinal cord. Kriya includes techniques to awaken a human's latent potential, inspire creative energy, and encourage the awakening of this energy within the system. This potential kundalini energy is described as residing in the general location of the sacrum.

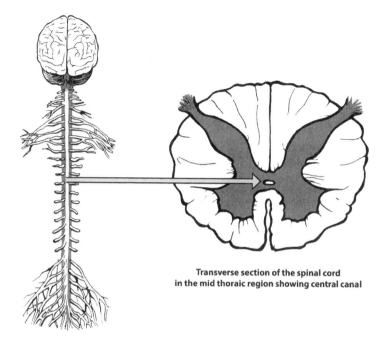

Transverse section of the spinal cord
in the mid thoraic region showing central canal

Figure 6.4. Central canal. Considered by some to be a
partial anatomical correlate to the sushumna.

logical, and spiritual processes in meditation can move forward with the
least resistance. To facilitate this proper posture, it can be beneficial for
the Kriya yoga practitioner to gain an intimate connection to the body
by understanding a bit about the anatomy and physiology of the spine
and skeletal muscles.

### Spinal Column
The spinal column is alive. It is not a collection of dead mineral depos-
its but in fact a column of living and breathing vertebrae that are connected to fascia, tendons, ligaments, muscles, nerves, blood vessels, and
prana. Treat it well, after all it is your backbone!

> *Maintain your spinal column as a column and not in arch.*
> GANESH BABA

The vertebrae are designed to transfer the weight load appropriately so that the back itself and particularly the spinal cord is primarily straight without kinks or torturous bends due to slouched posture. If properly aligned, the vertebral bodies manage weight well, with little stress or strain. Imagine that your body is suspended from a string coming up from the vertex of your skull into the sky, and your weight is balanced and gently transferred down your hips and into the ground through your ischial tuberosity, or sit bones, on each side of your pelvis. The goal here is to learn to balance the spinal column so that it is strong, resilient, and flexible.

This process helps develop a solid structure that provides a foundation from which to act. "Stay in your back body" is a phrase I first heard used by Manuela Mischke-Reeds, a Hakomi therapist, and I find it refreshingly practical and pragmatic. It describes maintaining a strong erect and alert posture that is balanced, flexible, engaged, and ready to act, but at the same time is in a deep state of relaxation and stillness. With time and practice of Kriya, one's posture also provides a resource for emotional stability as well.

Our spine consists of three sections: the cervical, thoracic, and lumbar vertebral bodies. They all have a slightly different shape and provide different functions. The cervical vertebrae make up our neck and are very flexible. They provide the direct support for our heads. Proper balance of the head on the cervical vertebrae is important. During certain aspects of meditation, the head is tilted forward and the chin is brought down toward chest while at the same time the cervical vertebrae are kept straight and aligned. This is part of the neck/throat lock, or *jalandhara bandha* (see chapter 9), and serves to flatten out the cervical curve, providing a slight stretch in that area of the neck.

The thoracic vertebrae protect our lungs and heart while at the same time providing support for our ribs, which need to be able to move up and down with respiration. The thoracic is the area of the spine that tends to become "hunched" for many in the modern age. Ideally one's posture is straight yet flexible and allows the ribs to hang fairly freely and move with each breath. But that movement becomes impeded as one hunches over. The goal of many of the physical exercises as well as the breathing exercises is to increase the thoracic space and the active volume used within the lungs for complete exchange of the air in the environment with our breath.

The lumbar vertebrae are the largest and sit on top of the sacrum. Each section of the spine has its own curve, and the lumbar is no exception. During sitting meditation it is often helpful to have a slight exaggeration of the lumbar curve because it helps with the stability of one's pelvic base and support for the spine. In general westerners do better sitting on a blanket or pillow so that their knees are just lower than their pelvis. This allows for a comfortable, ever-so-slight forward rotation of the pelvis, which provides a slight exaggeration of the lumbar curve and relieves stress on the diaphragm so that full respiration can occur. By placing one's hand over the lumbar area, the spine can be felt between the paraspinal muscles, two larger muscles on each side of the spine that can approach the size of one's biceps if one's core is strong and they are utilized regularly to sit straight. Ideally the spine is inside your back and well protected from the environment. Unfortunately few in today's world have strong paraspinal muscles.

In addition to these three sections are the sacrum and the coccyx. The sacrum is a solid bone that consists of five sacral vertebral segments that fuse together when one is a young adult. The sacrum is solid and connects to the pelvis, which itself is two bones that are held together in the front by thick ligamentous connective tissue and in the back by its connection to the sacrum. The top of the sacrum joins the last lumbar vertebra and together they contribute to the lower part of the lumbar curve. The goal in meditation posture is to maintain a slight exaggeration of the lumbar curve because keeping this part of the back "flat" or curved outward while sitting puts stress and strain on the system, in particular the diaphragm, which interferes with breathing. Note that the sacrum will rock forward slightly when the pelvis and lumbar curve are adjusted accordingly. The coccyx connects to the sacrum and is referred to as our tailbone.

## Pelvis

The pelvis is the base of one's structural support for any sitting meditation practice. It is made up of two bones—one on the right side and one on the left—that connect in the front through the pubic symphysis and in the back on either side of the sacrum at the sacroiliac joint. By developing proper posture, one's weight gets distributed evenly and solidly through the pelvis to the ground. A solid pelvis with strong core muscle development provides the structural support for meditative practice.

## Skeletal Muscles

There are three general categories of muscle fibers in the body: skeletal, cardiac, and smooth. We are mostly focused here on the skeletal muscles, those that allow us to move our limbs and torso through space. Cardiac muscles are concerned with the heart, and smooth muscles are involved with the various aspects of organ functions such as the walls of the blood vessels, intestines, and respiratory system, among others. Smooth and cardiac muscles tend to be involuntary and respond to their unique environments as our physiology changes from moment to moment. The body is both adaptable and incredibly resilient, changing as needed to help maintain homeostasis and balance.

Skeletal muscles on the other hand are under voluntary control and respond to intentional movements. These muscle fibers fall into two broad categories: fast twitch and slow twitch. Fast twitch muscle fibers tend to work quickly for short durations to help us with the intense bursts of energy needed to run, jump, and so on, but they fatigue quickly. Slow twitch muscle fibers enable long distance and endurance activities like sitting up straight for extended periods of time.

In general, slow-twitch-fiber muscles need to be used consistently to develop strength and stamina. In a slouched posture, the muscles needed to hold the spine erect are not engaged and therefore not activated or able to be strengthened. Many people experience the challenge of maintaining an upright posture for any length of time. One may become fatigued initially, feeling uncomfortable or cramping. As with any practice, the discomfort fades over time, as poise, grace, stability, and confidence build.

## MEDITATION POSTURE

To sit up straight means more than forcing the spine to be in a vertical line. Training the body to accept alignment requires attention to minor movements and small adaptations over time. In general, sitting with legs crossed or in lotus position provides the structural support for meditation, but sitting in a chair is also an option. If you're in a cross-legged position, do your best to provide enough support for your buttocks, thighs, and legs so that your posture is not a struggle to maintain. If you choose to sit in a chair, try to keep your feet flat on the floor with the sacrum toward the back of the chair, but the spine straight and away from the back of the chair.

In the beginning this task can cause fatigue. It is better to lie flat on one's back and take a rest rather than sit in a slouched manner. The body will conform to the most consistent patterns it is offered. Sitting in a proper posture as much as possible as you go through each day will surely result in rapid improvement.

If injury or pain prevent you from sitting this way, lying down can be an appropriate break in the beginning stages. The body will build resilience as you become stronger, and sitting straight will then be optimal. For the novice, however, lying down is not consistent with meditation. If you have trouble with strength or discomfort, consult with a physical therapist, trainer, health professional, or yoga instructor to get help in developing proper posture. Starting a simple, short but regular practice of exercise that you can do at home for five to ten minutes will make a very large difference.

The following steps will help you attain the proper posture each time you sit to meditate.

### ≪ Steps to Proper Posture

1. Sit straight and relaxed with a bolt upright spine to explore and feel the position with the most energy alignment. The muscles of the spine

and particularly the low back or lumbar spine should be engaged. The core abdominal muscles will also engage to assist the body in this position. Adjust the pelvis enough to feel the sit bones, or ischial tuberosity equally balanced on the mat, pillow, floor, or chair.

2. Roll the shoulders slightly back enough to feel a gentle squeeze between the shoulder blades and drop the tops of the shoulders gently down away from the head to create space in the neck. With time the shoulders will naturally move back and down with a stable upright posture, which helps to limit any slouching, maintains an open chest/heart area, and allows for full rhythmic respiration to occur. Bring the upper arms and elbows (at 90 degrees) close to the rib cage and then rotate your lower arms out slightly over your legs and allow your hands to gently drop to your thighs, palms down. In that position your arms should be fairly relaxed with minimal stress and strain on your shoulders, thoracic area, or diaphragm. Another option is to keep one's hands clasped in a relaxed fashion in one's lap.

3. Allow the sternum to rise with a deep inhalation and allow it to remain lifted. At the same time tip the chin down to reduce the curvature of the cervical spine and produce a slight pressure over the thyroid area. Imagine the vertex of the skull lifted to the sky and aligned with the antennae of the spine. This is not a rigid pose; rather it is active, engaged, and dynamic. The body may move to seek balance, as the mind becomes still.

4. It is important to check in with the shoulder blades, continuing to gently squeeze them together pressing the shoulders away from the ears and feeling the tip of the spine, the coccyx, close to the ground and well supported by the pelvis. Engage the belly slightly to keep it firm as a deep breath begins filling the pelvis and then the entire thorax or chest cavity, which holds the lungs, with breath. The abdomen will expand slightly as the breath begins to fill from the pelvic bowl upward, but it is not the main focus here.

5. Allow the face to relax, not holding any expression, and then slightly raise the eyebrows and relax the face in an expression of openness and curiosity. Relax the mouth with a soft smile and rest the tongue on the palate up behind the top front teeth. Relax the jaw and any other unnecessarily tense muscles in the body. In this way the structure of the body is used as a resource to contain the energy one is cultivating, refining, and redirecting.

The eyes can be open with the focus directed downward at a 45 degree angle toward a spot on the floor or wall or closed with the focus directed toward a spot slightly above the center of eyebrows without any stress or strain. This last option is mainly a focus of attention between the eyebrows and does not require the eyes to strain into an upward position.

---

When tuning in to the body, you are practicing a one-pointed focus, becoming more aware of yourself and sending attention to a specific area for a particular reason. The greatest gift we can offer ourselves or another person is our undivided attention.

## MICRO-MODULATIONS

As we begin to move down the road of practicing the four foundational exercises of Kriya yoga, we find ourselves in deeper states of reflection with an increasing awareness of more-subtle and refined levels of energy patterns in all four fields. We are now beginning to knock on the door of meditation and the synchronization of the foundational practices. As our awareness becomes increasingly focused internally, a new phase of creativity dawns upon the practice. Micro-modulation helps adjust perception of the subtle changes and awareness of the inherent power within the body.

Each field has its own exercises and its own range of micro-modulations to explore. Every individual has slightly different experiences with increasing awareness, integration, and transcendence.

## ❧ Micro-Modulations When Adding Breath to Posture

Now that you have spent time establishing your structural base, sitting with the ischial tuberosities in an upright, balanced, and flexible posture, it is time to move into breathing. Take a deep slow relaxed breath into the lungs, filling the spaces of the body, as you attend to the position of the tip of the coccyx and the vertex of the skull.

Make micro-modulations as you breathe in, sending attention to areas of the body. Where is the chin? Adjust it if necessary and breathe into the chest. What happens to your posture as the chest expands? Do you feel that a deep breath expands the body into a more relaxed position or a more rigid one? Are you holding tension?

What happens if you think about leaning forward one tenth of an inch with your whole spine as a unit, initiating movement from the top of your head while maintaining attention throughout the length of the spine? Breathe. Now do the opposite, leaning back, initiating movement with the vertex of your skull while maintaining awareness of your sacrum. First think about moving, then move. Try this again but only move one thirty-second of an inch one vertebrae at a time. Breathe. Each visualization exercise with regard to your spine should be accompanied by an inhalation, a pause, and an exhalation.

How do you experience your posture at these times? What do these micro-modulations teach you? You are always able to further refine your posture, further expand from top to bottom, side to side, and front to back. Can you expand the space between each vertebra at the same time? Observe and breathe. With each adjustment, allow time to reflect, visualize, and internalize the direction of prana in the body. Where we direct our attention, we will notice subsequent manifestations; where we direct breath, we will see life strive to meet it.

---

This is the fine-tuning of our antenna, the antenna that provides the reception for all the fields with which we will be interacting as we pursue the meditative process. As we breathe, reflect, visualize, and concentrate on these micro-modulations, we gain increasing somatic aware-ness and insight into the subtle effects of our prana, our life force, and how we experience and feel the change throughout our core being. It will also bring about greater changes in our ability to concentrate. The way to balance the mind is with the breath.

## INTEGRATING BREATH WITH POSTURE

Kriya is about experience. FEEL the breath. Learn to LOVE the breath. As the breath develops, it will create enough space to prevent thoughts from interfering. Notice where you feel your breath and how long you tend to hold it or gasp for it. Tune in to the pressure inside your body, the weight of your form, the immense power of each muscle that moves in unison to help the body breathe. Feel the temperature of the air as it is drawn into the nostrils, as it cools the upper lip or warms it upon its exit. Imagine pulling the breath directly up through your nasal passage-way into the frontal lobe of your brain, bathing the brain, and nourish-ing the universe inside. Conversely, you may also imagine breath filling the pelvic bowl, stretching the base of your spine so the sacrum spreads to each of its corners. Simultaneously, the muscles of the back are nour-ished by a fresh blood flow and oxygen.

The secret to integrating this experience is to allow yourself to drop in fully to the sensations and feelings that arise without resistance. Relish this feeling with curiosity as the waves of breath come and go. Direct breath to expand the rib cage in all directions, to the space behind the sternum and right up to the beginning of the front the neck. SAVOR the breath. What subtle changes do you experience as you shift your focus to the various areas of your thorax? Allow the breath to settle, becoming more subtle, yet purposeful; rhythmic, yet all-encompassing. As you move back and forth between micro-modulations and breaths, you cultivate a foundational weaving of verticalization (V1) with venti-lation (V2), becoming ever more graceful and grateful for the infinite expression of the human being as it aligns with Spirit and Nature. With time and practice your breath will begin to breathe you.

# 7

# Pranayama and the Cultivation of Joy

*It is all in the breath. Learn to love your breath;*
*it is your life's breath after all.*

Conscious awareness is key in developing and reconnecting to the Intelligence of Nature as expressed in our own biology. Our awareness coupled with our unique ability to develop conscious mindfulness is what enables us to fine-tune our experience of joy and makes us uniquely viable as a species. Worry, stress, trauma, apathy, and illness are all examples of ways our daily awareness is disrupted. We become disorganized as a pattern or body of energy and must work harder to regain balance. Yoga is the art and science that can help reduce the fluctuations and disruptions of awareness.

As discussed in previous chapters, the direct channel to making this possible is the practice of proper posture and pranayama, or breath control. Pranayama is the practice one uses to manage energies in the body and mind so higher levels of concentrations can occur.

*Breath control is mind control.*

Throughout childhood, we become aware of ourselves again and again; we are perpetually "reborn," so to speak, at new levels of development and curiosity. It is like awakening to our surroundings with a different perspective and envisioning ourselves in a new way. Where along the path to adulthood do we forget to explore our world with this natural curiosity? When is it no longer a miracle to see flowers bloom or watch the clouds in the sky? When we fail to perceive life with curiosity, our conscious awareness suffers and, after enough time, our bodies suffer as well. Perhaps people live with symptoms of pain or stress for so long because they are not connected to their bodies, and they forget to tune in to the subtle voice of intuition. Pranayama nourishes prana and builds strength for the integration of body, mind, and spirit.

## PRANAYAMA AS AN ART AND A SCIENCE

The word *Kriya* comes from the roots *kri* meaning "work" and *ya* meaning "Soul" or "breath." Therefore, Kriya yoga is the work done with the Soul's breath.[1] Breath-focused meditation is an ancient tradition that has evolved through many permutations over the millennia and deserves to be honored as a living tradition. As with any art form it can be detrimental to the practitioner as well as the art itself to become lost in rigidity, such as that found in many books written on Kriya yoga and pranayama that are acutely prescriptive in their directions and require rigid timing, counting, and particular movements. It is important to understand certain basics, but not to become rigid about their application.

Ganesh Baba himself was very supportive of the creative process and in fact referred to his form of Kriya yoga as "Crea," for "creative communion" or "creative integration." Although there are basic rules of the road for meditation, there is very little that is absolute. This book, once again, is a guide to help those who are searching for such a technique to begin to delve deeper within these guideposts on the path to further refinement of meditative practice.

In general, as long as the practitioner is proceeding with the basics—verticalization (V1), ventilation (V2), visualization (V3), and vibrationalization (V4), or posture, respiration, internal gaze (third eye), and mantra/inner sound—then one can expect to receive the pleasure and vibrancy of this practice. We all have the innate intelligence within us to go down this path. We just have to be still long enough to allow it to manifest. Remember, the "guru/teacher is within you."

Practicing pranayama in and of itself is an art and a science. There are certainly guidelines, and they do vary from one school to another. There is a consensus that the three energetic gate locks, or bandhas, of the throat, diaphragm, and the perineum are involved in most yogic schools of meditation. The bandhas are the group of three muscular diaphragms in the body that include the throat, abdominal diaphragm, and the pelvic diaphragm and they will be discussed in more detail in chapter 9.

In most pranayama exercises, there is generally a focus on inhalation, exhalation, and retention, but the ratios can vary. There are also multiple variations but sticking to a basic pattern until it becomes second nature is the most productive root practice.

Kriya yoga remains alive because its practitioners nourish, cherish, and honor it for the flow it provides; the routine, the simple techniques, and the insight toward joyful awakening. Learning the basic skills provides a foundation on which more complex skills can be built. Just as the child gradually integrates body awareness with small incremental steps, so does the conscious mind acquire greater expansion with meditation practice. This is the way with pranayama. It involves understanding that the automatic breathing controlled by the brainstem that sustains life is not the same as a conscious and directed breath. Beginning with a routine so one can comprehend the organization of breath assists the practitioner in remaining fluid rather than rigid and helps to keep the supple subtleties of this form aligned.

It is important to remember that the underlying goal in a breath-focused technique such as pranayama is to gain experience with the breath while remaining present in the body and playfully curious. Gaining mastery, one can begin to explore deep meditation and experiment with breathing rhythms in ways that affect awareness of the consciousness and Knowledge of the true intelligence inherent in Nature and Spirit. With the expansion of our lungs we become more awake to the intrinsically connected body, mind, and spirit.

The order in which to practice pranayama when first learning can be very important. Initially one wants to practice simple inspiration and exhalation. The initial goal is to develop the capacity to maintain a full regular, reposed, rhythmic respiration that is even in both effort and duration. It should be largely stress free and practiced without much strain and only with the appropriate erect sitting posture. Ultimately one can always be bolt upright and therefore always attuned and in practice no matter what life task is at hand.

Techniques have been developed to accelerate the learning process, particularly for the purpose of initiating one in the skills of meditation as opposed to simple relaxation or generic mindfulness. Development of pranayama can take time, and it is the accelerated path of this practice that Kriya presents. The practice of self-regulatory techniques can bring a sense of calm and decreased stress to an individual's overall system. With time there will be a deep sense of somatic relaxation and a decrease in anxiety, worry, and nervousness. The intention is that you will experience an increased sense of joy, calmness, and connectedness.

As one proceeds to engage with the breathwork techniques, one can expect both physiological changes and shifts in perception. One may experience an inner sense that one has arrived home for the first time. It is also possible that these or other feelings such as joy and grief can rise up and sometimes be overwhelming. Grief does pass with time, as it tends to transmute into compassion.

There can also be a sense of fear regarding mental stability as one experiences a more awakened state that is beyond "standard" reality. If thoughts arise like, "What is happening to me?" "This is too intense!" or "I can't take this!" it is best to sit straight, return to slow, steady breaths, and allow the intensity to subside. Of course, there comes a time when surrendering is essential if one wants to proceed. Remember that Kriya yoga is a process of energy management, focused on intentionally increasing conscious awareness. With practice one begins to get a sense of how life energy can be managed, moved around, and explored.

For practitioners who are psychologically and physically healthy and have an erect spine, and so on, the ability to engage in full relaxed respirations is more often safe than not and can be a life-changing experience. At some moments along the way it requires the courage to allow, release, and surrender to the flow. When one is facing trepidation, doubt, and fear of expansion it may be helpful to remember this art is also a science with many hundreds, if not thousands of years of human experience. Self-regulatory techniques are opportunities to grow and change and, of course, change can be uncomfortable at first. However, it is also during the beginning phases of this practice that one may have moments when the breath is full of the essence of prana and with each breath one can feel bliss and soulful expansion.

Breath, prana, and transcendence are all intimately related. Breath builds prana, which puts in place the foundation for growth and expansion. It is however, posture and a stable base that helps breath practices evolve exponentially. These practices are just like exercises used to cultivate any other skill. There are basic things to learn before knowing how to utilize them and move forward with more complex tasks. One skill builds upon another, and with each new level new awareness, perspective, and integration emerges from the new skills learned. This is like a craft where one has to learn how to use tools and the nature of the medium being used in order to master it. It is no different in Kriya yoga. Posture, breathwork, and concentration are all fundamental skills.

The breath is unique in that we have both voluntary and involuntary controls over it. We cannot hold our breath to the point where we would die, but we certainly can hold our breath to the point where we can pass out. Our breath is a direct link into the deep aspects of our brainstem, which controls our level of arousal and is a way we can encourage communication between the parasympathetic and sympathetic parts of our autonomic nervous system. It is a voluntary link that allows us to influence our overall state of awareness, consciousness, and stress management. In general, humans cannot easily adjust their rate of digestion or change their heart rate, but most individuals can easily adjust their breathing patterns and in turn the relationship with prana. This relational and embodied change will have a direct and immediate effect on awareness, attention, mood, anxiety, and cognition.

Breathing with prana, feeling prana in the breath, will guide the practitioner to a metaphysical continuum (the bio-psychic and intello-conscious fields) where the practice is further refined. Time is a mental construct, as demonstrated by Einstein's theory of relativity, and does not pass at the same rate for everyone. It is not important to focus on how long it takes someone to get to a destination with this practice, only that it is practiced in an ongoing fashion. Once we transcend what we think of as normal mode of time (beyond the speed of light), time loses its relevance and what exists is a perception in meta reality beyond the four-dimensional space-time continuum. This is the realm of prana, which transcends both. Our experience of the cosmos continues to shift as we learn from experience and build skills. Yogic philosophy sees prana as the quantum life energy that moves through physical space, body, and beyond. Michelangelo saw his sculptural work as breathing life into the stone he carved. One can think of prana in a similar way in that prana breathes life into the matter of the space-time continuum. It is prana or life that is depicted as passing from God to Adam in the Sistine Chapel's ceiling's "The Creation of Adam." Is it not?

In this chapter we will focus on some specific techniques to a greater degree of detail. It will be helpful to remember that these are all techniques that need to be experienced and embodied as Kriya is an experiential path. By carefully reading the detailed instructions, studying the illustrations, and if necessary exploring some other resources such as yoga teachers with training in pranayama techniques or online or DVD videos (see appendix 2 for a list of some audio-visual online resources), even new practitioners should be able to experience a shift in physiology and perspective.

## PRANAYAMA PRACTICE

A pranayama practice begins by bringing awareness to the breath as often as possible.

When do we typically consider breath? Perhaps when we are holding it, gasping for it, yawning, or realizing it is somehow interrupted. Feeling the bodily experience, the "embodiment," of all of the exercises in this book is of the utmost importance.

Let us begin with reflecting on the difference between our usual waking state of breath, which is largely unconscious in its flow through the day, by contrasting it with conscious breathing. By conscious breath I mean just that, breathing while at the same time bring your conscious awareness of the moment to the task of each inhalation and each exhalation.

The basic breathing techniques are noted in the list below. Some are slightly more complicated than others and require further explanation, but most are fairly simple and self-explanatory. We will be exploring them in more detail in this chapter and hopefully with time you will not only learn them but master them as well. In yoga most breathing exercises occur through the nose, unless otherwise specified. By gaining some mastery one can then begin to explore the art of meditation by exploring breathing patterns in ways that affect our awareness and consciousness. Once this exploration begins, we can move forward in a more intelligent and compassionate fashion by unifying our body, mind, and spirit and connecting it with joy.

## BASIC BREATHING TECHNIQUES

- Inhalation (*puraka*)
- Exhalation (*rechaka*)
- Retention (*kumbhaka*)

- Full yogic breath (regular, reposed, rhythmic respiration)
- Ocean breath (*ujjayi*)
- Jet breath with relaxed inhale (*kapalabhati*)—also known as breath of fire or shining skull breath
- Abdominal breathing
- Vacuum breath (modified *uddiyana* bandha)
- Alternate nostril breath (*nadi shodhana*)
- Kriya Breath or the Balance of prana with aprana *(kevala kumbhaka)*

Remaining consistent with the practice and developing awareness is key in cultivating a life alive with consciousness. It is important to recognize changes as they occur, to be present in your shifting, but to also remember that no matter how deep a meditative state one obtains or how deeply one may merge with all that is, there is a silent master, witnessing. With time and deeper levels of meditation this silent witness becomes ever more distant. It is only in *mahasamadhi,* or the conscious leaving of the body, where the egoic self completely recedes.

The various different breathing techniques are further described below and we will begin to actively work with how to use them to engage in meditation and energy management. Should you prefer a slower and gentler progression, refrain from jet breath, vacuum breath, visualization, and mantra exercises, as these promote a more rapid growth. As we move forward please remember to always sit up straight.

## *Inhalation* (Puraka)

Inhalation itself is structured into three phases. The first phase is initiated by the engagement of the diaphragm and the filling of the pelvic bowl. The abdomen stays firm as the inhalation of air with prana begins filling up the torso from the pelvic bowl up into the abdomen and then into the ribs and upper chest and eventually to the clavicles. Bring awareness to the bodily experience of breathing.

The second phase is to attend to the ribs as they begin to expand in all directions, the sternum lifts to meet the chin, the chin lowers slightly to straighten the cervical spine, putting slight pressure on the thyroid area, and the shoulders relax so the clavicles may find a balance like a balance scale.

The last phase of inhalation is to attend to the upper chest where you feel the air come in and fill in the space just above the clavicles as your shoulders move slightly up and gently back and then come down with exhalation. During inhalation the spine continues to lengthen both from the vertex of your head toward the sky and from the tip of your coccyx down into the earth. It is also helpful to maintain a toned abdomen and offer your attention always to a straight, relaxed bolt upright spine.

### Exhalation (Rechaka)

Exhalation should also be smooth, relaxed, and reposed. It does not help to become so short of breath during pranayama that you gasp for air. Ideally exhalation is just as controlled as inhalation. The chest should not be allowed to collapse on exhalation. As one's practice advances, exhalations become longer than inhalations but again not so long that one gasps for an inhalation. Although inhalation is what keeps us alive, it is only with effective exhalation that proper inhalation can occur.

### Breath Retention (Kumbhaka)

Pranayama exercises include inhalation, exhalation, and breath retention. It has been said that retention is the goal of pranayama. Retention is an intentional interruption of inhalation and exhalation by voluntarily withholding breath. It is thought to be the essence of prana and energetic control. Retention requires training of dynamic breath ratios in order to build strength in the body and create a dynamic and active practice. In the beginning there will be only brief retentions, but with time the body and mind become more trained to hold the breath a little longer without negative effects. The length of retention is not a contest. Stay within the realm of comfort. Once again you do not want to gasp for breath at the end of retention when the lungs are full. You should still be able to engage in a slow controlled exhalation. There does come a point where the practitioner may experience spontaneous breathless states, corresponding with deep contemplative states of unity and this is different than voluntary retention.

Breath retention can come at the end of an exhalation when the lungs are empty (*bahya* kumbhaka) or at the end of an inhalation when the lungs are full (*antara* kumbhaka). Breath retention after exhalation can also be thought of as breath suspension. This is also what is done as part of vacuum breath. When breath retention happens spontaneously (*kevala* kumbhaka), the lungs are neither full nor empty. This is the breathless state, a moment of ultimate balance of inhalation and exhalation, when states of transcendence begin. This cannot and should not be forced!

It is important to note that the rhythm of the breath is more important than the amount of air that is retained. The retention should end before the individual has to gasp for breath. After it ends, exhalation should proceed with a slow rhythmic and complete exhalation without any abrupt jerky motions. This is something that comes with practice and experimentation. With time retention will leave the practitioner feeling prana, the essence of breath throughout the body.

Full breath retention allows a delicious savoring of deep oxygenation that is felt throughout the body. At the same time the practitioner uses the various energetic gates/bandhas (explained later in this chapter) in the torso to help contain the prana, which contributes to the meditative experience through interaction with the vagus nerve of the parasympathetic nervous system (see chapter 10). It can also be used to direct the breath toward a specific spot in the body for release or expansion or when deep moments of transcendence occur. It is also of note that breath retention works best on an empty stomach, particularly if full inhalation is being retained. On the other hand, a light meal or a nice cup of chai often goes hand-in-hand with a deep relaxed meditative session (see appendix 3 for an excellent chai recipe).

## Full Yogic Breath (Regular, Reposed, Rhythmic Respiration, or R4)

The basic yogic breath in this form of Kriya is a full regular, reposed, rhythmic respiration. This is referred to as R4. R4 is the backbone, or the workhorse of breath-focused self-regulatory techniques. This type of respiration can be varied by coupling it with various forms of retention and by varying ratios, rhythms, and depths of relative inhalation and exhalation. Initially the goal is to be able to have a full rhythmic respiration that is reposed, rhythmic, and relatively deep and soothing, and ideally, this pattern of breath becomes one's regular conscious pattern through each and every day. To reinforce this idea we sometimes say, "R3 + 1" in order to put emphasis on the importance of using R3 (reposed, rhythmic respiration) regularly (+1). With time a very, very subtle yet full and deep breath develops with the practice of breath focused meditation. It is the conscious breath of Kriya that is precursor to the breathlessness point, and is on the path toward Self-Realization.

When first practicing this technique we calmly but fully inhale through the nose and then exhale for a relatively equal duration and force. If there is some anxiety and stress, the exhalation can come out through the mouth and with a slight sighing sound, as one's shoulders drop back and down, although most yoga breathing is done through the nose. Of course, maintaining proper posture and alignment during these exercises is of the utmost importance regardless of what technique you happen to be using at the moment.

This is an excellent exercise to begin to acquaint oneself with the beautiful and divinely nutritious nectar of the breath. All of the breath-focused self-regulatory techniques/pranayama described in this book will bring added value to one's psychospiritual development, particularly if one can foster a deep love and appreciation for the wonders of breath.

### ❮❮ R4 Practice

1. Begin the practice of R4 by filling up from the pelvic bowl with breath. Many people have been taught abdominal breathing, but this tech-

nique differs in that we are building on the initiation that starts in the pelvic bowl, then bringing the breath up to expand the ribs from the front, the sides, and the back, and then moving up to the upper chest above the clavicles and feeling the breath come all the way up to the neck at the Adam's apple/thyroid gland.

2. Maintain firmness in the abdominal muscles at all times rather than allowing the abdomen to engage in flaccid expansion. Straight posture is important with this and all breathing techniques as the diaphragm muscle connects to the low back and cannot function properly in these exercises without straight posture.

3. At the same time, add retention with inhalation for a couple of seconds before allowing a slow, rhythmic, controlled expiration, aided by the abdominal and intercostal muscles. All the while remain engaged in a fluid posture that is bolt upright, with shoulders back and down and with a sternum that is high and close to the chin (see figure 7.1).

4. Count to a number between two and eight during each inhalation and exhalation to help train the body to retain the practice and commit it

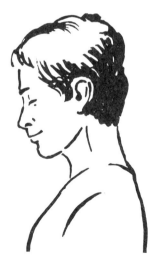 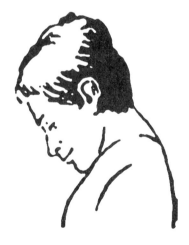

Figure 7.1. Chin position during meditation. The example on the left is a mild version of the throat lock (jalandhara bandha) used during deep meditation. The version on the right shows a more pronounced throat lock, which is used during breath retention.

to muscle memory. Be consistent with what feels right to you and try to initially have the in and out breaths be the same length. The ratios below represent the pattern of inhalation, retention (on inhalation), exhalation, retention (on exhalation) and are written in this order. Full exhalation is what most people need to learn first. Taking a deep breath in during inhalation is easier to learn as most everyone has experience with that. Please know that these ratios are just patterns to play with. With time the breath will become very subtle and find a relative balance in all its component parts. That will occur over time as you develop a more intimate relationship with your breath.

———————————————

Some patterns of commonly used ratios when beginning are 1:1:1:0, 1:1:2:0, and 1:2:2:0 if tolerated you can try 1:4:2:0 which will move you toward an experience of true retention. To further clarify, if you were going to use the 1:2:2:0 ratio as an initial counting method, you could use counts of 1:2:2:0, 2:4:4:0, or 4:8:8:0. For example, 4:8:8:0 is a count of 4 on inhalation, said silently (one, two, three, four), then a count of 8 for retention, followed by a slow exhalation to a count of 8, and no retention on exhalation so one would go right back to inhalation and repeat the process. This does not mean you should count during this process as a practice. The idea of counting is for illustration purposes at the beginning and not for routine practice. Remember, it does not have to be perfect! With time these patterns become easy and natural and you might try adding a couple of seconds of retention at exhalation as well, such as a 1:2:2:1 ratio. This will increase the strength of the lungs.

The above ratios are slanted toward exhalation and retention of the inhale as those are the most out of synch in many. The next focus is more on the even-handed nature of a meditative breath where the inhales and exhales are more even. The ratios to play with in this area are 1:1:1:0, 2:1:2:0, and 2:2:2:0 ratio followed by the addition of retention on exhalation 1:1:1:1 and 2:1:2:1. Once again these are not rigid parameters but exercises for experiencing the breath in different ways so that one's own innate respiratory intelligence is gently woken after years of slumber and shallow breathing practices.

If I had to pick one of these to master first for deepening meditation it would be one of the two following patterns: 4:4:8:2 or 4:16:8:0. These will give you some sense of longer retention on inhalation and slow exhalation, which ultimately expands respiratory capacity and helps with accessing deeper states slightly quicker. If you have a watch with a second hand it can help you see what this feels like. For example, in the 4:4:8:2 ratio the inhalation and retention on inhalation are both 4 seconds long. The exhalation is 8 seconds. If 8 seconds for exhalation in this ratio is too long at first, you can try 6 seconds. The retention after exhalation is 2 seconds long. Try it a few times and see what it feels like. The inhalation should be more robust compared with the slower exhalation as you are moving the same amount of air in half the time.

As expertise develops, various other ratios can be explored. Retention times can be extended but not to the point where one needs to gasp for air. In my experience it is best to go with dynamic creativity once the basics have been embodied. It should also be noted that the ratios will change some within any given practice session. Remember this is your life, your breath, your journey, and your flow. All of which are inherently creative processes. There are other variations as well but sticking to a basic pattern until it becomes second nature is the most effective root practice.

Breathing this way neutralizes anxiety and increases alert attention. For accelerated spiritual growth, it is recommended that breath retention be included as early in one's practice as feels comfortable.

· · · · · · · · · · · · · · · · · · · · · · · · · · · · · · · · · · · · · · · · · · · ·

## Flow

Another way to conceive of the form of Kriya breathwork is as a CREAtive dynamic flow of poetry in motion. Learning to loves one's breath goes a long way here. You will learn to follow the movement of posture, breath, prana, concentration, and awareness as they ebb and flow while dancing with each other. With time and capacity, the delicate all-pervading essence of Kriya breathwork will move in and take over the show. Your job at that time is to abide in the creative glow of Kriya as it unfolds within you and around you.

There are many explanations and formulas for yogic breath. Pranayama exercises are extremely helpful in retraining the respiratory system to help it find its inherent roots. After years of trauma, anxiety, pollution, and poor posture, the respiratory system is struggling to maintain a balance. Is it able to keep us alive? Yes, it is. Is it able to gain a foothold and help us toward further human evolution? Not unless we help it. Kriya yoga is all about reinvigorating the respiratory system through posture and concentration so that it will allow the integration of inhalation and exhalation in an embrace of ecstasy.

So how do you accomplish this? If you do some research on the various pranayama techniques you will find a multitude of suggestions on how to practice them. The bottom line is that your relationship with your breath will change as intimacy develops. Although it is helpful to begin with a fairly even inhalation and exhalation with brief retention, with time you will develop a different relationship with each type of breath. You'll begin to understand it and feel it and intuitively gravitate toward one type over another, depending on where you are moving in your state of conscious awareness.

Please, please, please do not turn this into a formulaic exercise. Kriya yoga breathwork is alive. It is the creative force of Mother Nature, reaching and connecting with the awareness of Spirit coming together to allow experience of the infinite, the nondual reality.

• • • • • • • • • • • • • • • • • • • • • • • • • • • • • • • • • • • • • • • • • • •

I would like to add here that some lines of Kriya do not give these suggestions for the breath, allowing it to develop on its own over time. It is my experience that a little pranayama goes a long way for it provides a reeducation, so to speak, of the respiratory system. One can think about it like learning to play a sport. If baseball was the sport the skills required would include throwing, catching, batting, running, and sliding, to name a few, as well as understanding the rules. Once the basics are embodied one can "play ball." Kriya breathwork is similar in that pranayama wakes up our respiratory system teaching it new patterns, which quickly allows for the deep patterns of R4 (R3 +1) to move in and replace the unconscious shallow breath. It is for this reason that pranayama exercises are of benefit as ultimately deep meditative states rarely employ rapid breaths. In fact, the deepest states of meditation correspond to the spontaneous breathless state where the air exchange is so subtle it is hard for an observer to detect it.

## *Ocean Breath* (Ujjayi)

Ocean breath is a breathing technique that includes a gentle restriction at the back of the throat to reduce the amount of air coming in and out of the lungs. The restriction of breath causes a soft sound in the back of the throat, like whispering loudly or blowing on a mirror to fog it up. It can also sound like ocean waves and can be generated both on the inhale and the exhale. The larger the volume of air and the quicker the movement the louder the sound. This breathing technique provides a number of additional benefits—one being the vibration that can be felt in the back of the throat/pharynx and nasal area/nasopharynx—and can vary in intensity.

The area that is restricted is in the throat and is called the glottis (vocal cords), part of the larynx or voice box, which is a muscle that changes its shape as we engage in these activities. The area of the nasopharynx (just above the pharynx) is also involved as the air is traveling through that area as well. It is the area of the nasopharynx that is not far from the brainstem, the third ventricle, the pineal gland, and the nuclei of the vagus nerve, which is intimately involved with the meditative experience. Ideally, this breathwork technique is done in a full, regular, reposed, and rhythmic respiration. It can be practiced by coupling it with various forms of retention or ratios, rhythms, and depths of inhalation and exhalation. The initial goal is to perform full rhythmic respiration that is deeply soothing.

## *Jet Breath with Relaxed Inhale* (Kapalabhati)

Jet breath with relaxed inhalation is a lively way to play with the art of pranayama. This is also a very important component of the accelerated path of Kriya. It consists of a series of intentional, short respirations that begin with a rapid, robust exhalation through the nose followed by a relaxation of the diaphragm to allow breath to flow in on its own. The pressure differential that allows for the relaxed inhalation is set up by the rapid forced exhalation. This breathwork helps to "detox" the lungs by exhaling residual air and carbon dioxide from the deeper crevices in your lungs that do not typically get evacuated during normal breathing, allowing for more oxygen to enter on the longer inhalations that follow in R4. It is also useful in further refining concentration after a prolonged meditation session if one wants to reenergize in order to reenter deeper meditation again and extend the session. This technique is also energizing before a meditation session and can help beginners and advanced students move more quickly into a deeper meditation at any time. This is the only pranayama technique in this book that allows for inhalation through the mouth, although the nose is preferable. It is very important to remember that inhalation happens on its own upon relaxation. Jet breath does not include any active assist in the inhalation process it is an exercise that focuses on rapid forced exhalation. A jet breath exercise can be found below.

## ᠈᠈ Jet Breath Exercise

In this pranayama exercise the abdomen needs to relax to the point that it may initiate and passively absorb inhalations quickly (see figure 7.2). This breath can be done as a series of one breath after another in rapid succession or in a series of three breaths, one rapidly following the other, with a slight pause between each group of three. This can be an intensely energizing and activating practice and it is important to remember proper posture. Please note that jet breath does not incorporate ocean breath technique.

To begin the exercise, sit up straight, shift your attention to the

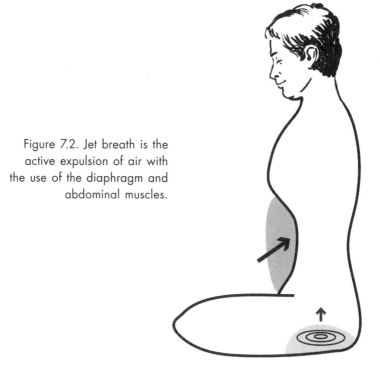

Figure 7.2. Jet breath is the active expulsion of air with the use of the diaphragm and abdominal muscles.

abdomen, where pressure is exerted with the abdominal muscles from the navel area back toward the spine, forcing an exhalation through the nostrils. The exhalation is coupled with engagement of the *mula bandha*, or root lock, which is an increased tone of the anal sphincter and perineum area (see chapter 9).* Pay attention to the shoulder blades, which will move back toward your spine, as well as a slow subtle rhythmic extension/flexion movement of the lumbar spine. This can be facilitated by bending the elbows with hands up toward your chest and pretending you have chicken wings as you pull your shoulder blades back toward your spine and flexed arms follow as you exhale.

This coordinated effort provides a subtle rocking motion of the body while jet breath is actively engaged. As you rock your pelvis

---

*To make this jet breath exercise more powerful pair it with movement of the low back and mild shoulder movement (see pages 121–24).

forward and your lumbar curve increases, forcefully exhale. Then as you passively inhale relax back to a straight position and repeat the process. This is an active rhythmic pattern of rapid pressured nasal exhalation with passive inhalation coupled with an active yet subtle rocking movement of the pelvis and lower back. When you exhale, bring your shoulder blades together toward your spine and then relax them when you inhale. The final piece to this exercise is engaging the root lock. It can be engaged throughout the exercise but especially during the exhalation process. During this exercise the thorax will also be in active movement; however, it is the abdomen that is engaged and active on exhalation and relaxed on inhalation, which occurs automatically. (For more on jet breath see page 158.)

---

This combined exercise is often a difficult one at first. Practice each piece by itself and then integrate them together. This exercise energizes the body, mobilizes prana, and provides strengthening of the core muscles and respiratory system while at the same time priming the system for deeper meditation. This is a coordinated rhythmic movement that is challenging to learn but once learnt becomes second nature. The length of time one is able to engage in this practice will depend upon the physical fitness of your lungs. It is also important to note this exercise can quickly lead to lightheadedness, even in just three to five breaths. If this should occur, the practitioner is encouraged to return to slow relaxed respiration. The number of exhalations depends on what one can tolerate. Some individuals practice for five or ten seconds and others can do it for much longer.

It should be noted here that more is not better, and there can be complications if one gets carried away with this exercise and does it for too long. This should simply be utilized as an energizing technique to the point of benefit without becoming lightheaded or agitated.

### *Abdominal Breathing*
In addition to posture, it is essential to understand another factor before going forward: abdominal control. In Kriya yoga we consistently

return to and improve upon both. While posture is the initial focus in Kriya yoga, understanding abdominal control with pranayama is also key because the abdominal muscles must stay engaged at various levels. The savasana and abdominal breathing exercises in this section along with the vacuum breathing exercise in the next section can help to expand one's experience and understanding of abdominal control. These exercises can help one to explore retention on inhalation with abdominal muscles that are engaged to provide counter pressure to the expanding lungs and lowering diaphragm. This provides solidity and strength and further helps to contain prana. It is through active engagement of the abdominal muscles that improved respiration is activated.

## ❦ Abdominal Breathing in Savasana, or Corpse Pose

The savasana pose can be a deeply restorative pose that can help one to become familiar with one's body and breath. There are many descriptions of proper positioning available but in general, a practitioner lies on their back, sometimes with some support for the head and shoulders, although any head support should be thin, so as not to add to any neck strain. The goal is for the body to be able to relax deeply. When positioning oneself, there is a goal of symmetry. This is not always possible based on age and what one's body can tolerate. Sometimes this pose goes along with a body scan exercise where there is a progressive relaxation of the muscles moving slowly upward from the toes to the head with alternating contraction and relaxation of each body part in a systematic fashion. There are many recordings available that can guide one through this exercise as many variations exist.

During savasana, one allows one's breath to "just be" and does not attempt to direct it in any fashion. As there is not much to "do" in the pose it can be quite challenging. But on the other hand, entering it with a beginner's mind can lead to a deeply nurturing experience.

Although the savasana posture is not typically part of Kriya yoga, it can be helpful for beginners in breathwork to explore the use of the abdomen with the breath while in this pose, so it is included in this book. When in this position, place the hands, palms down, gently over the abdomen and then observe the breath. Placing a small rolled-up towel on the abdomen can give you a greater sensation of weight on your belly as it moves up and down, making the action easier to observe. One can also engage in slightly deeper breaths and as one is supported by the floor, it is sometimes easier in the beginning to explore different rhythms of breath in this way. This position is certainly not suited for other pranayama techniques, but a gentle abdominal breath pattern can be very soothing as one moves through the body scan exercise described above.

## ≪ Abdominal Breathing Kriya Style

Many individual's first breathing exercise is what is referred to as abdominal breathing. By and large R4, a full, regular, reposed, rhythmic respiration is a more complex form of abdominal breath. We have looked at various breath rhythms and now look more at the how to aspects of this essential breathing technique. As one begins to breathe in, the diaphragm contracts, moving downward toward the abdomen and pushing it out slightly while at the same time the thorax, or chest cavity, expands. Allowing this first step to happen can be very challenging for those who have spent much of their life wearing tight cloths and trying to hold their abdomen in, which can limit the natural expansion of the abdomen and pelvis areas. In fact, as the full abdominal breath begins the abdomen moves out and you want to be aware of the pelvic bowl as it begins to fill while at the same time maintaining engagement of the abdominal muscles.

The second phase of the abdominal breath occurs once the abdomen has expanded somewhat and the chest cavity begins to expand with the ribs moving up and out in the front, sides, and back. At this time the shoulders move slightly back and, in Kriya, the back of the

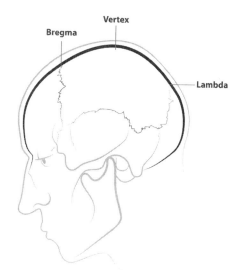

Figure 7.3. Bregma, vertex, and lambda.

skull rises slightly as the chin tilts down to meet the sternum, which is rising as the air continues to fill the chest. In Kriya, we do not want the head tilted back toward the sky. If anything, we want the vertex, or a point between the vertex and the *lambda* point (see figure 7.3), to be the highest point of the head as the head tilts forward, lengthening the cervical spine and lowering the chin toward the sternum.*

The third phase does not include a lot of air exchange compared to the abdomen and chest areas, but nonetheless it is filling the last bit

---

*This is not the first time we will be discussing tilting the head slightly downward during various exercises. As you will learn later in chapter 9, there are certain areas of the body with a tendency to focus more energy than others. In Indo-Buddhist meditation traditions, these areas are referred to as chakras. The three points identified in figure 7.3— bregma, vertex, and lambda—are all associated with the crown chakra. When meditation teachers speak about the "fontanel," they can be referring to any of these three areas, depending on the their particular lineage and the specific focus or techniques they are refereeing to. Anatomically speaking, bregma is the remnants of the anterior fontanel, the soft spot that closes in infants, and lambda is the remnant of the posterior fontanel that also closes shortly after birth. As one tilts the head forward in the neck/throat lock, bregma moves forward and down and lambda moves forward and up, so that the vertex becomes the highest part of the skull. Depending on one's individual anatomy, this highest spot can be closer to lambda. However, throughout the text, we be referring to the vertex as the highest point.

of the lungs with air, and with some effort one can feel the air rise up slightly above the clavicles. Now is a time when you can try retention if it feels right. Then it is time for slow and rhythmic exhale.

This exercise can be done in a very mild or more rigorous fashion. By rigorous I am referring to moving toward maximum capacity of air coming in, but mild versions are also helpful. In fact deeper states of meditation occur with very subtle breath. What the deeper, more active respirations provide is exercise, stamina, strength, and a repatterning of one's usual breathing routine so that deeper natural and more subtle rhythms can rise to the surface, which we can then ride on our way to changes in our awareness.

### Vacuum Breath (Modified Uddiyana Bandha)

Vacuum breath is a form of retention that uses the diaphragm lock also known as uddiyana bandha (see figure 7.4) to allow for the

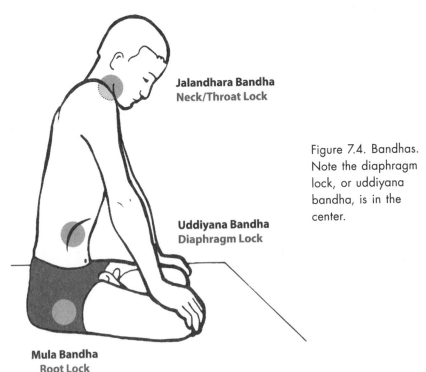

**Jalandhara Bandha**
**Neck/Throat Lock**

**Uddiyana Bandha**
**Diaphragm Lock**

**Mula Bandha**
**Root Lock**

Figure 7.4. Bandhas. Note the diaphragm lock, or uddiyana bandha, is in the center.

engagement of the abdominal muscles, which helps a new practitioner become better acquainted with respiration in general and breath control specifically.

## ❄ Vacuum Breath Exercise

1. Begin by taking a deep inhalation. Then engage the abdominal muscles to aid in a deep and complete exhalation. Slowly and gently at first, but gradually a little more forcefully, attempt to push out the air in your lungs for a full exhalation. The goal is to push a sizable amount, if not every last bit, of the air out of your lungs by forcefully engaging your abdominal muscles and diaphragm to assist in an exhale.

2. Suck the abdominal wall in, further pulling it closer to the spine without inhaling any air. This is done by attempting to inhale, but not allowing air in.

3. While keeping the air out at full exhalation, try an abdominal pumping action, a sucking in of and then relaxing your abdominal wall without any air exchange. This retracts the abdominal wall into the abdominal cavity, allowing one to gain control over musculature not typically used in this fashion. In addition, this "false inhalation" also provides a deep and rhythmic massage of inner organs.

4. After this retention of breath, quickly relax and release the abdomen as you allow yourself to inhale. You want to experience a swooshing sound as the air from the outside environment rushes in to fill the pressure gradient in your lungs through your nostrils, thus the "vacuum" effect. This is not necessarily a routine exercise, but it does help with repatterning/reeducation of the respiratory system in general. It is helpful at the beginning of training and it is also something that helps the advanced practitioner return to a deep state of meditation when one is interested in exploring further and wants an additional assist. With time you will hopefully think of it as an old friend.

---

## *Alternate Nostril Breathing (Nadi Shodhana)*

Alternate nostril breathing can be a very soothing and regulating breath practice. Traditionally it is used in many yogic meditation practices to help balance the right and left energy patterns in the body.

## ⫷ Alternate Nostril Breathing Exercise

Typically, the thumb and ring finger are used alternately to close one's right and left nostrils as part of this breath practice. And as with all breath exercises, posture should be upright and straight.

1. Get into a full, regular, reposed, rhythmic respiration. To move into the alternate nostril breathing, bring the right hand up to the face and use the right thumb to close the right nostril. Inhale in a slow, reposed fashion through the left nostril.

2. Close the left nostril with the right ring finger and pause for a brief moment of retention with both nostrils closed.

3. Then, leaving the ring finger on the left nostril, lift the thumb from the right nostril and exhale.

4. Now inhale through the right side, again in the nice slow rhythmic fashion, and then once again close the right nostril with the thumb and hold both nostrils closed for a brief moment. Then release the left nostril and slowly exhale through it. This is one complete cycle, and it can be done a few times or more.

---

This is a simple, soothing technique, but while it's particularly helpful in reducing stress and anxiety, it is not necessary for Kriya. It is included here for you to experience, and I recommend that you try it. The more experience you can have with breath the better.

## KRIYA BREATH OR THE BALANCE OF PRANA WITH APRANA (KEVALA KUMBHAKA)

This is a difficult subject to put into words but is something you will recognize when you experience it. It is sometimes referred to as the breathless state. In general, it is the meeting of prana (the inhalation) and aprana (the exhalation) that brings the practice of pranayama to its apex. There are many ways to conceptualize this idea. It references the meeting of the more material-based energies of Nature with the more ethereal energies of Spirit. In India, these two are often referred to as Shiva and Shakti but can also be viewed as masculine and feminine, yang and yin, or positive and negative. It is the coming together of the vibratory nature of polarity that allows for creation. It is the initial vibration of the Absolute, the pronov, The Word, which gives rise to the material universe from its nondual nature. The two aspects of the prime polarity of Spirit and Nature come together once again in the breath at the moment when prana and aprana meet in the breathless state. It is this balance of breath that ultimately allows for the release or rising of kundalini, which is discussed later on.

The goal of the pranayama exercises above is to prepare the respiratory system to become immersed in the deep quietude of a very subtle almost breathless state which occurs when several physiological parameters are met. If you remember, breath control equals mind control. Once the body is thoroughly oxygenated through more rigorous breath exercises it begins to slow down. Initially respiration remains full although the rate of air exchange becomes more and more subtle to the point that it becomes barely perceptible. The goal of starting with jet breath and moving to full regular reposed rhythmic respiration is to prepare the system to quiet down and allow for and even encourage sensory retraction to take place. As V1 to V4 integrate, a deep sense of joy begins to pervade one's body, mind, and soul. This is what Lahiri Mahasaya referred to as the "after-effect poise of Kriya." It is the beginning of deep states of meditation that are induced by the more active practices of Kriya, which shift our physiology to the meditative state of awareness. With practice and time these breathless states of Kriya become easier to and easier to enter. This is the Kriya breath of Kriya yoga, the joining of prana and aprana in perfect balance.

## DEVELOPING YOUR PRACTICE

Developing a pranayama practice takes consistent discipline. Practice, practice, practice is the refrain. If one follows the exercises as outlined a new relationship with the breath will develop. Once you experience a sense of joy from the breath you will be well on your way although like any intimate relationship it will need to be nurtured and cherished. If neglected it will take a little more effort to bring it back around. You may forget Kriya but once you have touched the essence of Kriya, Kriya will not forget you.

Once you are comfortable with slow R4 breathing, move on to practicing retention. Initially you'll want to try retention after inhalation for a brief pause, and then continue with a nice full exhalation as previously practiced. Once you have a sense of working with retention begin more focused work with jet breath and then vacuum breath. These techniques will form the basis of infinite ways to move deeply into the realms of Kriya breathwork and hence toward moments of stillness and deeper insights into the nature of Kriya and Nature herself.

Developing of a full pranayama practice can take many years, although the benefits can start almost immediately. These combinations of techniques have been developed to accelerate the process and effects of meditation. Those who are interested in a softer, slower, and gentler progression of skills should continue along the lines just explained by slowly adding retention after expiration. It is the addition of jet breath and vacuum breath, coupled with further visualization and mantra exercises, that accelerates the process, and we will explore all of these exercises in an actual Kriya practice session at the end of the next chapter.

# 8

# Refining the Techniques and Creating a Kriya Yoga Session

---

*To work with your mind, you'll have to be patient; you'll
have to cultivate a collaborative working relationship
with yourself and your posture and your breath,
which ultimately controls the mind.*

---

You may have noticed that this book seems to have its own silent mantra that is repeated throughout, and were it said out loud, it might sound something like this: "Sit straight and it will come." While it is true that a sound physical structure is the core of Kriya yoga technique and practice, there are many subtleties that go into refining one's practice. Now that we've gone over some of the basics, we will look in more detail at other aspects of developing a solid and mature Kriya yoga practice as they apply to the four Vs (see figure 8.1 on page 118 for a reminder).

For each of the four Vs there are both macro and micro-modulations that help adjust our perception of the subtle changes within the body (see page 88 for more on the use of micro-modulations). For each of the primary Kriya yoga exercises in the V1 through V4 sections of this chapter you will find a range of micro-modulations to explore.

# Kriya Yoga
## The Basics

| V1 | Verticalization | Posture | Spinal Awareness |
|----|-----------------|---------|------------------|
| V2 | Ventilation | Breath | Reposed Rhythmic Respiration |
| V3 | Visualization | Third Eye | Sensory Retraction |
| V4 | Vibrationalization | Mantra | Inner and Outer Sound |
| | | Meditation | |

Figure 8.1. The Four Vs.

## VERTICALIZATION (V1)

As we have discussed, proper posture is the first step in this form of Kriya yoga. Learning and maintaining proper posture is easy for some but fairly challenging for others. This section reviews some of the general ideas and practices to help develop and maintain a proper anatomical upright posture and a strong structural base. Think of this section as a guide. With the one possible exception of lumbar mobilization the physical practices in this section are more like a menu to pick and choose from. No two physical bodies are the same. Therefore, the physical practices to improve posture while similar will have variations in the routine. The goal here is to listen to your body and consult with a professional if you need additional guidance. This section could be a volume all on its own. The choice was made to keep it simple in the tradition of Ganesh Baba's teachings. You are encouraged to explore other hatha yoga sources to obtain additional insight into the brief overview below. These physical posture based practices are meant to be explored with the goal of improved strength and resistance in one's own posture.

In this section we will also review the concept of mudras which are physical positions of various parts on the body to effect changes in energy patterns. Mudras are included here as they involve the physical body.

### Limb Limbering

In this accelerated form of Kriya practice Ganesh Baba stressed what he liked to call "limb limbering" (see figure 8.2). In fact, he was a great advocate of physical activity and would often get out his cymbals and begin to dance and sing. Limb limbering is an all-encompassing, generic term that Ganesh Baba used to describe physical exercise, strength training, flexibility, and resilience.

There was no strict regimen with regard to frequency or specific repetitions in this aspect of Kriya yoga training. In fact, the only requirement of this line of Kriya was a straight back and straight breath. It has been my experience over the past forty years that Ganesh Baba was absolutely correct. Some level of physical fitness is helpful in order to be able to sit still in meditation, and sitting still on the outside is an important factor in being able to reach deep stillness on the inside.

That said, the physical fitness aspect of a meditative yoga practice is very flexible and depends on what an individual needs to work on. It is for this reason that this book is intentionally loose with regard to

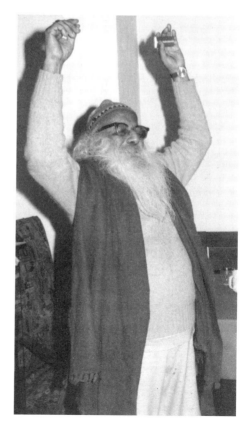

Figure 8.2. Ganesh Baba limb limbering, circa 1986. (Photo by Michelle Cruzel.)

the formal practice of the physical asanas or exercises. However, it is important for a serious student to pursue hatha yoga, tai chi, qigong, or physical therapy or visit a gym, get a personal trainer, practice the Five Tibetan Rites, or just develop their own routine. Slouching while sitting is not an option; neglecting limb limbering isn't either. Find a reasonable routine that focuses on your weak points and practice that routine every day. Maybe you have two routines that you alternate. The most important part is developing a strong physical core that is flexible and resilient so that you can practice the techniques of Kriya yoga. You will be surprised what five minutes of focused work on physical postures will do for you. Remember to always get guidance from a trained practitioner or teacher before taking on physically taxing activities that are new to you.

Two particular exercises that Ganesh Baba did stress regularly was that of lumbar mobilization and shoulder shuffling. These exercises are of utmost importance in that they activate the central nervous system, engage the respiratory system, and anatomically open up the thorax to allow for a full, deep respiratory experience while at the same time engaging the shoulder girdle and improving posture. These two exercises themselves are not sufficient to develop a strong, resilient structure, but they are essential in activating the breath engine of Kriya yoga, which becomes a breath and prana reservoir.

Before we move on to the details of these exercises, we must take a moment to review the anatomy of the spine, as it will help clarify terms as we move forward. Anatomically speaking, spinal "flexion" is when one bends forward or curls up in a ball, in the fetal position. Spinal "extension," on the other hand, refers to the motion of the spine when one leans backward. You can also open your heart center with this extension by slightly opening the arms and looking up toward the sky.

When Ganesh Baba taught Kriya he referred to the exercise below as "lumbar flexion." Although there is some flexion involved, it is more of an extension exercise and therefore the name has been changed to "mobilization" as that more accurately describes the task at hand.

Ultimately, it is the strength, resiliency, and flexibility of the spinal column that we are focusing on: the strength to maintain the spinal column as a column and not an arch, and the flexibility of structure that allows blood, lymph, central spinal fluid, and neurological transmission to flow through it. Motion is the essence of life. Rigidity, stiffness, and brittleness make it harder for life to move forward. The more we care for our spine, the younger and more joyous we will feel!

## *Lumbar Mobilization*

Of course, we begin by making a point of focusing on the straight and upright spine. This, however, does not mean it should be rigid or stuck. In fact, we expect the spine to have its normal, natural curves, and it is these curves that balance the spine and provide the structural support needed for the body to function optimally. With lumbar mobilization we increase the flexibility and strength of the spine and help the body relax more fully into its foundation.

The technique is fairly simple after a little practice. Begin with a slow and gentle rhythm. With each exhale during jet breath include a slight forward-rocking motion of the pelvis that exaggerates your lumbar curve. On inhalation the lumbar area straightens as the pelvis rocks slightly backward (see figure 8.3 on page 122). As you do this you will be engaging a number of postural muscles of the spine as well as your diaphragm and your perineum. The engagement of your perineum/pelvic diaphragm root lock helps contain the energy generated in a meditation practice of breathing techniques. We will discuss these locks, or bandhas, in a little more detail later in this chapter.

Remember to keep your posture erect and your shoulders back with each exhalation. Figure 8.3 shows the hands resting on the legs. This is a fine position for mild to moderate jet breath with lumbar mobilization. In more active moments of practice the forearms should raise up off the thighs, no longer touching them. This allows for more rigorous shoulder involvement and lumbar movement. This exercise can be a slow and steady pace or one that is a little more lively.

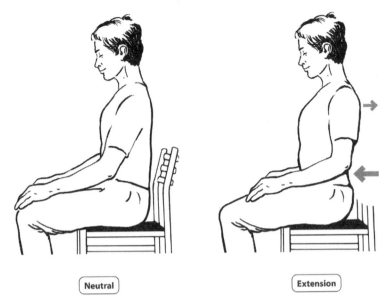

Figure 8.3. Lumbar mobilization.

Often, you will be using shoulder shuffling and lumbar mobilization at the same time in a synchronous fashion with jet breath. This is all a bit complex at the beginning and sometimes feels completely backward. You may want to try practicing each aspect (jet breath, lumbar mobilization, and shoulder shuffling) separately and then begin to combine them. Once you get the hang of it this technique it can be used at any time to refocus and energize your meditation. If you become distracted or lose interest during meditation and want to reengage and reenter the deeper and slower breathing states, these techniques can be very useful. This practice should not be overdone and it is helpful to have a guide while learning how to synchronize and utilize these techniques. They are without exception powerful and effective tools.

## Shoulder Shuffling

In this section were going to talk about general awareness of shoulder posture as well as some passive stretching and then move into the active use of our shoulder girdle to complement lumbar mobilization and jet breath.

Before sitting for meditation, it is beneficial to do some stretching or movements to help the body relax into a strong, stable foundation. "Shoulder shuffling," as Ganesh Baba referred to it, is one such exercise that is easy to do and helps open the rib cage, thorax region, and chest. It also assists in increasing one's awareness of the spine and helps to maintain its erect posture. If our shoulders are not anatomically correct, our respiration is significantly impaired.

Our shoulder blades, or scapula, are designed to glide over the rib cage. During the day, many of us experience our shoulders creeping forward and upward and the scapula naturally follows. Rather than being on our back where it belongs, the scapula almost ends up at our sides. This markedly impedes the ability of the ribs to move with each respiration.

Our arms are usually down by our sides or bent at 90 degree angles in traditional work settings as we lean over computer screens, drawings, books, etc. Other "higher" primates spend time in trees and use their arms in markedly different ways, which allows for an expansion of the thorax and the need for strong muscles that hold the shoulder girdle, including the scapula, intact. As few of us do much in the way of climbing with our arms in regular activities, the engagement of exercises that include our arms and shoulder blades is important to allow our thorax to open for complete and full respirations.

One simple activity you can do as you sit down to meditate every day is to lift your arms over your head and stretch upward. Pretend you are climbing a ladder with your arms as they move up and down. Try and imagine that you can feel your weight as you pull yourself up rung by rung. Now try and stretch your arms out to the side with the shoulder blades back. Be creative, slow, and mindful. Explore your limits and get help to learn about properly expanding your limits of flexibility and strength in this area.

When your arms are at your side be mindful of keeping your shoulders blades back and creating an open space within your chest. With an inhalation bring your shoulders up toward your ears. Pause. Move your shoulders back and down as you gently exhale. Feel your shoulders

relax and let go. Repeat this until you feel your shoulders have had sufficient movement to keep them flexible and then continue your breath
practice without exaggerated shoulder movement. Be careful with your
shoulders as they are a complex joint and injuries can take quite a while
to heal if they get strained or injured. Learning to keep an open thorax
with shoulders back is one of the best ways to strengthen the shoulder
girdle and help prevent chronic-use injuries.

When one is practicing lumbar mobilization, the arms and shoulder blades can be used actively to aid in the general exercise. As one's
lumbar curve is exaggerated, the lower spine bows forward. See if you
can bring your shoulder blades back toward your spine while slightly
exaggerating the lumbar curve. Bend your elbows bringing your hands
up and pretend your flexed arms are wings in a way. With each rhythmic movement forward as your spine bows, your pelvis rocks forward.
Let your chest open and expand while you bring your shoulders, shoulder blades, and elbows around your torso slightly toward the back in
a gentle, slow rhythmic fashion. This will also include some extension
of the mid-back thoracic area. Ideally each bowing extension of your
spinal column is occurring at the same time as jet breath exhalation.
There will be a concurrent engagement of your perineum, as well as
your abdominal muscles and diaphragm, which forces air out of your
nostrils. As you slowly and rhythmically straighten your spine and
relax your abdominal muscles, your lungs become filled automatically
and are ready for the next forced exhalation in conjunction with the
combined contraction of your perineum, abdomen, and diaphragm.

## Hatha Yoga Poses

The following yoga poses are included to be an optional guide for limb
limbering as they offer many benefits to improving physical strength,
flexibility, concentration, and connection to breath. Any daily routine
of a few physical movements will improve these areas so think about
choosing exercises that will serve your body so that your body, mind,
and spirit can engage with joy in meditation.

It is best to work with an instructor to get a felt sense of these postures and to ensure safe and effective practice. A gentle introductory hatha class can be a helpful way to explore how breath and movement can work together. However, there are many resources online to help get a better understanding of these poses. *Yoga Journal* maintains a very nice website that has pictures and descriptions of these and other poses. There is no need to become proficient in all the yoga postures included here, but if you are physically able to engage in some of them, they can be very beneficial.

These postures are arranged in an order that can be followed one after another if such a routine is desired. It is also good practice to pick a few to focus on from time to time so that a deeper understanding of each posture is internalized. The first six poses are fairly easy and can be beneficial to both beginners and seasoned practitioners.

Sun Salutation also known as *Surya Namaskar* is another exercise that incorporates connected movement in an organized flow. There are many online resources that can offer clear steps to practicing it, but, again, working with a skilled instructor to cultivate a felt sense of the postures is best.

## ≪ 1. Mountain Pose (*Tadasana*)

- This pose is used as a foundational standing pose as well as a transition pose between other stretches. It is one that can be useful throughout the day to practice deep breathing and feel embodied alignment. It is also the way to begin a walking meditation where one is walking while using sound/mantra outside in a secluded area. Because of its use in meditative practice, we are including a more detailed description.
- Stand up straight with your feet together and find a connection between your feet and the ground that is supportive. Heels are usually slightly apart with the big toes close enough to touch. The goal is to feel balanced, relaxed, and slightly taller. This happens as you begin to gently shift your pelvis back and forth until you find a balance in the middle.

- The next step is work with the torso and shoulders. Taking a full breath, be mindful of the shoulders going up and back and the shoulder blades moving toward the spine.
- Next balance your head over your pelvis and feel the top of your head get taller as your feet firmly plant on the ground.
- Follow this with a few deep breaths as you relish the alignment of your body and breath.
- Being more aware of posture while standing or sitting helps build body memory. Become acquainted with the back body and the spine and use this pose to practice standing meditation as well as a starting position for walking meditations.
- For a walking meditation try maintaining an erect posture as you walk and breathe rhythmically while repeating an inner mantra. If you are away from others you may want to try using your voice and develop a deep rhythmic resonating sound/mantra that has a cadence you find enjoyable. Try it, you will enjoy it.

## ❰❰ 2. Plank Pose (*Phalakasana*)

- This pose is like the top of a push-up and helps develop core strength. Practice holding for one minute while breathing. Then consider moving into Child's Pose.

## ❰❰ 3. Child's Pose (*Balasana*)

- Kneel with knees slightly parted and chest resting upon thighs. This is an excellent stretch for the spine.

## ❰❰ 4. Cat Pose (*Marjaryasana*)

- Come onto all fours and arch the spine to round the thoracic spine. Combined with the cow pose, this posture provides improved spinal flexibility.

## ❰❰ 5. Cow Pose (*Bitilasana*)

- Come onto all fours, curve the spine, and move the back of the head toward the tailbone. It is good practice to alternate between cat pose and cow pose.

## ⫸ 6. Sphinx Pose (*Salamba Bhujangasana*)

- This is a beginner backbend. It starts with lying on your belly. Your elbows are placed below your shoulders with the forearms parallel in front of you. You make a slight arch in your back as the upper body lifts from the floor. Once again we are working on strength and spinal flexibility here.

## ⫸ 7. Downward-Facing Dog (*Adho Mukha Svanasana*)

- This pose can be done independently or as part of sequence called Surya Namaskar, the Sun Salutation. Facing the floor, with hands planted shoulder distance apart and feet planted hip distance apart, lift your bottom into the air to create a V shape with the body. This provides a deep stretch for the extremities as well as some core strengthening.

## ⫸ 8. Staff Pose (*Dandasana*)

- Come into a seated position with back and legs at a 90-degree angle. This helps strengthen back muscles and also can open the shoulders and chest. It also provides the starting point for the next exercise.

## ⫸ 9. Head-to-Knee Pose (*Janusirsasana*)

- Begin in seated staff pose and move forehead toward knees. This posture enhances flexibility.

## ⫸ 10. Bridge Pose (*Setu Bandha Sarvangasana*)

- Lying on your back with feet planted hip distance apart, lift your hips off the floor while using your shoulders as a base. This is likely the most physically challenging pose on this short list and is best explored with a teacher. Once again, we gain some flexibility with this pose as well as core and upper body strength.

## ⫸ 11. Knees-to-Chest Pose (*Apanasana*)

- Lie on your back, bring your knees to your chest, and hold them in place with both arms to relax the low back. This can be deeply relaxing allowing for breath movement and gravity to help with alignment.

## ❦ 12. Corpse Pose (*Savasana*)

- This pose is intended to promote deep relaxation in the body. It is typically practiced at the end of a yoga class but may be a pleasant place to begin as well.
- Lie flat on your back and place one hand on the chest and one on the abdomen to feel the full rise and fall of the belly as you breathe. Become more conscious of the body and simultaneously more restful in this position. It should be noted that lying down is not conducive to learning meditation. That said, the corpse pose/savasana can be deeply restorative at the end of a hatha yoga practice or other exercise.

---

### Five Tibetan Rites

Another routine that is helpful is the Five Tibetan Rites (5TR), many descriptions of which are available online. The Five Tibetan Rites is a series of five hatha yoga–like exercises practiced twenty-one times in a particular sequence. They may have their origins in a form of Tibetan yoga. The rites are known for their physical, mental, and spiritual benefits. The only exercise we do not recommend in this group is the spinning exercise, as it is not needed in Kriya and can bring about vertigo in many people over forty years of age. However, the core strength provided by the 5TR is quick and impressive. Teachers of this technique recommend twenty-one repetitions but seven or eight is a good initial goal and may prove sufficient based on your fitness level.

### The Bow (Gratitude Pose)

Technically a bowing motion can be a yogic posture or an asana such as Child's Pose, but in this case we are focusing on bowing from the sitting position. In many traditions bowing often initiates from the standing or kneeling position, but when seated in meditation it is natural to move forward in the act of bowing with the same intent.

The bow can provide a lot of support for the structural, respiratory, and psychological components of a contemplative's meditation practice. The physicality of bowing has the psychological component of surrendering to something greater than yourself or your own universal Self. In addition, it provides a physical stretch for your spine, potentially activating the parasympathetic system through the innervation of the dura mater, the covering of the brain and spinal cord, with the cranial nerves. Try this before and after you meditate.

## Mudras

Mudras are specific positions, poses, or gestures that have different meanings in a variety of Eastern traditions. In Kriya yoga there are five specific mudras to explore: *maha* mudra, Shambhavi mudra, yoni (*jyoyi*) mudra, *khechari* mudra, and namaste mudra. They are physical in nature and exert influence over the body and mind. Maha mudra is more of a physical hatha yoga exercise and focuses on spinal flexibility and the breath. Shambhavi mudra refers to eye movement toward the third eye. Yoni mudra, on the other hand, provides a structure for a specific finger and arm placement that provides additional support for the visualization and vibrational aspects of Kriya yoga and is utilized once one's posture and breath are firmly rooted in stabilized practice. Khechari mudra is for advanced practitioners who have few worldy responsibilities. Namaste mudra is ubiqutous in Eastern culture but can be very powerful if practiced with an open heart and intention.

### Maha Mudra

Although Ganesh Baba taught maha mudra, only a few practiced it extensively. Maha mudra is certainly helpful in developing some aspects of pranayama. In fact, ultimately maha mudra, if done correctly, is a wonderful exercise for pranayama and flexibility that tends to focus on spinal flexion. If one decides to practice maha mudra, the breath is the most important aspect and with time, the posture and movement will come. While some lines of Kriya yoga make maha mudra a primary practice for Kriya yoga, Ganesh Baba's teachings focused more on engaging in limb limbering first, pranayama second, and then as visualization (V3) and vibrationalization (V4) are engaged, moving into what

Lahiri Mahasaya's after-effect poise of Kriya. It is my experience that Ganesh Baba's techniques provide quick results with or without maha mudra, although including maha mudra can certainly be synergistic.

Eve Neuhaus, another one of Ganesh Baba's faithful students and author of *The Crazy Wisdom of Ganesh Baba,* describes maha mudra in the following way:

> To perform the maha-mudra, sit on the floor and place the left heel on the perineum. The right leg is extended [straight ahead] at a right angle to the body. Inhale deeply and slowly concentrating on the third eye between the eyebrows. Visualize a brilliant tube of light, the sushumna, running through the center of your body from the top to bottom and exhale as you slowly bend forward to clasp your right foot firmly with both hands. Hold your breath as long as you can. Release your right foot and sit up bringing the right knee to the chest while inhaling deeply. Exhale while sitting, releasing the energy into the ground. Inhale deeply, drawing energy from the earth and repeat the process twice more on the right and three times on the left with the right foot on the perineum, and finally three times at the center, clasping both feet.[1]

Here's another version of maha mudra (see also figure 8.4):

## ≪ Practicing Maha Mudra

1. Sit on the floor and place the left heel on the perineum.
2. Pull the right knee into the chest with both hands, so that the right abdomen feels pressure.
3. Inhale and retain the breath while stretching the right leg out in front and bending forward to clasp the right foot with both hands.
4. Release the right foot and sit up pulling the knee back to the abdomen and exhaling slowly and deeply.
5. Switch legs and repeat the process before moving to both legs at the same time.

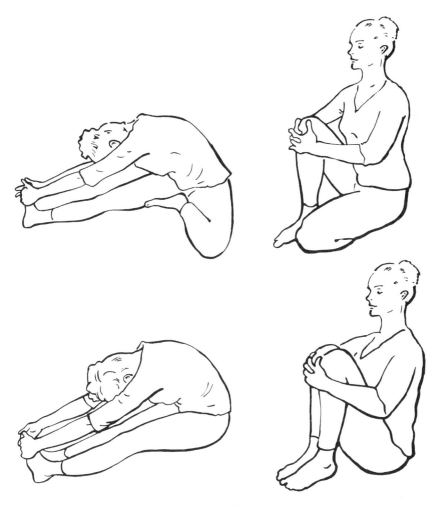

Figure 8.4. Maha mudra.

The above are examples of just two different versions that vary to some degree. The important aspects of this practice are the spinal stretch and having the additional pressure on the abdomen when one's lungs are full. For beginners it may be helpful to use two breaths for this mudra. The first is inhaling when one is sitting up and holding the right knee against the abdomen and chest and then exhaling. This is then repeated when one inhales and then forward bends and holds the foot and retains the breath. Exhalation then occurs as one returns to the upright position. Thus, there are two periods where the breath is retained and pressure is added to the abdomen. One can choose to do the right side, the left side, and then the center and repeat in that pattern, or one can do a series of three on the right, three on the left, and then three in the center. The symmetrical pattern of alternating right and left and then doing the center is preferable.

## Shambhavi Mudra (Third Eye Gazing)

Shambhavi mudra, or third eye gazing, is an exercise in attention training as well as movement and stabilization of the eyes (for more on this see the sections on visualization (V3) on pages 72 and 141).

## ❰❰❰ Practicing Third Eye Gazing

1. Focus your mental attention on the third eye without consciously shifting your gaze. There is often an unconscious slight movement of the eyes toward that space between the eyebrows. This is perfectly natural and there is no need to resist.

2. As the attention becomes stronger and the third eye begins to show itself one can often feel a pull on the eyeballs that easily and without strain directs them to the center of the third eye. Allow this to arise. Shambhavi mudra is the term that describes this ultimate direction and focus of the physical eyeballs to the spot of the third eye.

3. A few very important additional adjustments of the facial musculatures can add a lot to this mudra. The first is to make sure you are not furrowing your brow. The second is to raise the eyebrows slightly as that helps with the third eye focus. Last allow a slight smile to emerge in another subtle movement that contributes to the meditative practice. These three minor adjustments are uniquely powerful and should not be dismissed or overlooked.

## Yoni (Jyoti) Mudra

This technique assists one in sensory retraction, or pratyahara. Its goal is to decrease the sensory input through the eyes, ears, nose, and mouth, which helps beginners focus on the internal sound. Historically this technique was only given during initiation. In the current age it has been published in books on Kriya yoga as well as online. Due to its broad availability it is included here.

## ⪻ Practicing Yoni Mudra

1. Place the thumbs gently over the opening in the ears, close the eyes, and rest the index fingers on the ridge of the lower bony orbit of each eye, ever so gently pulling the eyelid down (see figure 8.5).
2. Place the middle fingers on each side of the nostrils to provide closure as needed and the ring finger and smallest finger above and below the lips to assist in closing the mouth.
3. Bend the arms at the elbows and hold the elbows at a 90-degree angle from the body so that they are parallel to the ground. In this way, there is no restriction of the thorax and therefore full rhythmic respiration can proceed.

---

The effect of this mudra is to provide a markedly different experience of the inner world in short order, as it is helps to accelerate one's experience of inner light and sound. The breath is practiced in a traditional full yogic breath fashion but with retention on inhalation using the root lock/mula bandha. Some lines of Kriya suggest that one should

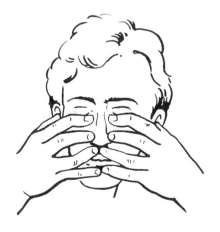

Figure 8.5. Yoni (jyoti) mudra.

spend a long time on this technique. As with all techniques, however, once it is mastered, repetitive use is not typically needed, but occasional use can be helpful for a quick tune-up if needed.

## Khechari Mudra

The khechari mudra is a technique where one moves the tongue back into the pharynx behind the uvula and up into the nasopharynx area. This is a powerful technique that takes one into deeper meditative states. There are different opinions on this mudra within the Kriya community. Some feel it is essential and others do not. It is a challenging mudra to learn but just by placing one's tongue on the upper roof of the mouth at the junction of the hard and soft pallet give one can an idea of the shift that can occur in awareness when the tongue moves deeper into the skull. That said, Ganesh Baba was very clear that this technique was only for those who were renounced or retired and no longer engaged in householder activities, otherwise regular practice of the mudra could make it difficult for a practitioner to engage in the activities of daily life.

## Namaste Mudra

The intent of the namaste mudra is to bring a message of deep recognition of the Spirit that is within. This simple gesture is a way to take the energy from your meditation with you throughout the day as you have the opportunity to greet others on your journey by acknowledging that same divine energy within them.

### ≪ Practicing Namaste Mudra

1. Bring the palms together in front of the chest with fingers pointed upward.
2. Take a slight bend at the waist, as well as in the neck, as you make eye contact with another person and slowly exhale with the greeting "Namaste" or alternately bend remaining silent and greet or thank the person with eyes and heart. It can also be used at the beginning or the end of meditation or prayer.

## *Micro-Modulations in Verticalization (V1)*

We're always able to further refine our posture, to further expand from top to bottom, side to side, and front to back. Micro-modulations with posture are made as you breathe and send attention to different areas of the body. Each time you do this, inhale, pause, and exhale. Where are your shoulders? Adjust them so it is easy to breathe into the chest. What happens to your posture as the chest expands? Does the deeper breath expand your body into more relaxed position? Where are you holding tension? Can you expand the space between each vertebra at the same time? Can you become taller vertebrae by vertebrae? How about becoming taller by imagining your crown moving toward the sky while your coccyx moves toward the ground? What happens with a slight adjustment in the lumbar curve? Changing the height of your pillow or where you are touching the seat of your chair can make a significant difference in your posture. Try some variations. As you become more accomplished and your posture improves you may find further adjustments are helpful. The goal is to be able to sit with ease and grace while being as straight as possible. Observe and breathe.

Above are just some examples of micro-modulation for posture. They are all slight adjustments to posture that are also experienced in the breath. How do you experience your posture at these times? What do these micro-modulations teach you? The idea of micro-modulation applies to all aspects of Kriya including the mudras and exercises discussed above.

## VENTILATION (V2)

We have already spent a good deal of time discussing the breath, and all of those practices are part of V2. The following section includes deeper exploration of the breath through the bandhas, which function as energy gates for prana. By including these practices in meditation, one learns how to concentrate the prana of the breath within the body and hold it there in a more concentrated form.

## *Bandhas*

Bandhas are active processes of engagement with various muscular diaphragms in the body that when activated provide containment for the prana/energy that is generated during pranayama techniques. They are often referred to as gates or locks because they wall off, to some degree, the energy in the torso for optimal use during meditation.

There are four main bandhas that engage the practice of energy containment: the neck/throat lock (jalandhara bandha), the diaphragm/abdominal lock (uddiyana bandha), the root lock (mula bandha, see figure 8.6), and the combination of all three of these bandhas used simultaneously (maha bandha). To engage the bandhas, certain muscle groups, or diaphragms, are activated for various effects. They include the so-called vocal diaphragm (jalandhara bandha), the abdominal diaphragm (uddiyana bandha), and the pelvic/perineal diaphragm (mula bandha).

### Neck/Throat Lock (Jalandhara Bandha)

The jalandhara bandha, or neck/throat lock, is put into action in its complete form during breath retention, either after inhalation or exhalation.

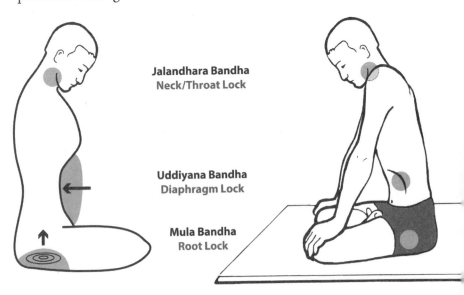

**Jalandhara Bandha**
**Neck/Throat Lock**

**Uddiyana Bandha**
**Diaphragm Lock**

**Mula Bandha**
**Root Lock**

Figure 8.6. Three bandhas.

It locks the respiratory process down to some degree, allowing the retention to deepen physiologically and energetically. This technique begins by slightly bringing the chin down/bending the head forward while keeping the neck straight, which exerts some pressure in the Adam's apple area where the thyroid gland is. The chin moves down toward the sternum and on a full inspiration the sternum moves up toward the chin. As a practitioner gains more experience with retention, they will find that keeping their hands on their knees and locking their arms for a period of time can add an additional component of stability. This often requires the shoulders to move up slightly. Once the breath has been retained to a point that feels comfortable, the practitioner gradually releases the breath. This bandha is also used in a modified form without retention in conjunction with ocean breath during R4 as a way to slow the breath and feel its subtle vibration as it goes through the airway passages.

Both the neck bandha and ocean breath involve the deep throat muscles that are part of the pharynx and the glottis that are involved in the control of sound and air going in and out of the lungs. It is these muscles that are being engaged here during a vocal throat bandha or ocean breath.

To engage the neck bandha, make sure your posture is straight, elongate your spine, and tilt your head slightly forward until you feel a slight pressure around your thyroid area. You want to feel the cervical part of your spine lengthen and the natural curve slightly flatten. Your breath will cause the upper part of chest to rise toward your chin. Engage the muscles in your throat and constrict them slightly to provide some resistance as air passes through the oropharynx and nasopharynx. It is the slight constriction of the throat and the slight pressure on the Adam's apple/thyroid that contributes to the oceanlike sounds that can occur on both inhale and exhale. This technique helps slow the breath down further by providing some resistance. It also straightens the cervical spine slightly to help with energetic flow and provides some additional vibration in the back of the throat and the nasopharynx, which is the airway between your nose and your throat. The nasopharynx is in very close proximity to the brainstem/medulla oblongata, the seat of the autonomic nervous system. Activating this area has a profound influence on our awareness and state of consciousness. Another structure close by is the fluid filled third ventricle, which has the pituitary gland near its front end and the pineal gland on its posterior side. These structures, considered by some to be the deepest part of the third eye, are referred to in Kriya texts as important areas of focus, and in yoga they are known as Brahma's Cave, or the seat of consciousness within the human brain. This can be an area of focus during V3, visualization with the mind's eye for more advanced practitioners.

## Diaphragm/Abdominal Lock (Uddiyana Bandha)

The abdominal bandha was described to some degree in the discussion on vacuum breath. You may recall that during this abdominal and respiratory exercise the lungs are emptied by quickly and forcefully exhaling—or slowly but firmly exhaling—as much air as is possible using the abdominal muscles. The abdominal bandha is engaged by keeping the lungs empty of air (retention on exhalation) and then moving toward an inhalation but not actually allowing any air into the airway at the point of the throat lock. This raises the diaphragm and sucks the abdominal wall in without allowing any inhalation of air. At this point, there can be a rhythmic pattern of this false inhalation, followed by relaxation without any air movement in or out of the lungs. The practice ends by relaxing the retention, allowing a full breath to enter on its own as the pressure differential is relieved and a swooshing sound is heard as the air rushes in. This is a practice in its own right as well as something to use as part of R4. In R4 it would be used briefly at the end of an R4 cycle after a full exhalation. At that time, the diaphragm bandha exercise of sucking in the abdomen can add additional appreciation of prana during the cusp of entering deeper meditation.

## Root Lock (Mula Bandha)

The root bandha is a contraction of the muscles in the perineal area. This can be slightly different in males and females but in general occurs as constriction of the perineal muscles that initially can focus solely on the anus but with time also includes the rest of the perineal area. This can be best experienced by engaging the musculature as if you were stopping urination in midstream. Having some engagement of the root bandha during Kriya yoga meditation can be helpful for maintaining posture in general. In particular it provides additional stability and strength for the lower back. Try it and see if you can notice a change. Its primary purpose is in the management of prana as well as encouragement toward the waking of kundalini.

## Combination of the Three Locks (Maha Bandha)

*Maha bandha* is the term used when all three of the above bandhas are applied together. These locks or muscular diaphragms separate various regions of our body and are engaged in order to gain control of one's energy or prana flow from area to area, allowing the practitioner to manage their pranic energy. The root and neck bandhas for example, lock the upper and lower ends of the spinal column maintaining the pranic energy generated in between those areas, preventing loss of the energy to the ground or the sky. The use of the maha bandha occurs during breath retention on exhalation. It is not part of retention after inhalation as the lungs are full and uddiyana bandha cannot be engaged in the same way. During R4 with retention after deep exhalation maha bandha can also be engaged and allow one to easily move into a few false inhalations of vacuum breath adding some additional energy to the meditation. This is a good time to emphasize the combined use of just the upper and lower bandhas, the neck lock and root lock, which are ideally engaged together when retention on inhalation occurs.

Bandhas are uniquely capable of nourishing energy centers and balancing prana throughout the body. Once a practitioner has learned to manage their energetic bandhas in the torso they will benefit from being able to contain the prana that contributes to deeper meditative experiences. Deep retention of breath serves other purposes as well as one may direct the breath toward a specific part of the body for release and expansion. Retention should be smooth and flow from breath to retention to breath easily without abrupt or jerky movements. Breath should not be withheld to the point that the practitioner must gasp for air. It is also best to practice this on an empty stomach as the internal organs will benefit from an internal massage with deep breathwork.

Although much of meditation is an energetic process the physical components such as posture, respiration, and the various bandhas affect both the physical and the energetic aspects of our being. Right about now all these little details may seem a bit daunting and overwhelming, but after a little experimentation the process becomes quite intuitive and can add a lot to one's practice at various times. It may be hard to believe but a little practice of jet breath and vacuum breath will allow all these other variations such as retention and the various bandhas to come about quite naturally. These processes are all hard-wired into the nervous system and just need a little activation so that they can take off and lead the way.

## *Breath and Direction of Prana*

With time and practice, directing prana, breath, or energetic attention to various parts of the body will become easier. Such practices can help open one's heart with compassion, relieve pain, or relax one's bronchi if stress from panic or mild reactive airway difficulties are present. In addition, focus can be directed to the fontanel. In fact, some lines of Kriya focus almost exclusively on the fontanel, which has many of its own benefits and experiences for deepening meditation. As these are all energetic experiences time and practice is needed to appreciate the differences here. That said many meditative traditions use the fontanel as the main focus. It is my opinion that focusing first on the gyral center, or third eye, and then on the fontanel allows for quick progress along this path. This is the way that was taught by Ganesh Baba.

## Micro-Modulations in Ventilation (V2)

We've already talked about various ratios to try when exploring inhalation, retention, and exhalation. You can also explore the edges subtly with the various bandhas and observe any subtle changes with your breath. See what happens if you lean slightly forward while you're employing retention on exhalation with all three bandhas engaged. What happens as you lean forward slightly and/or make your arms slightly more stiff when you engage in false inhalations? (For example, see the person on the left in figure 8.6 on page 136.) What happens if you take in a small amount of air before retention on inhalation? How does that feel compared to retention after taking in as much air as you can? What is it like to engage the neck and root bandhas on full breath retention versus breath retention without the bandhas? Always remember to keep the abdominal muscles somewhat engaged even during retention with inhalation. How do different breath rhythms affect your third eye or the rhythm of primal nodal vibration, repetitive sound, or mantra? The combinations are infinite and once one has a stable routine that is working for them additional doors will open suggesting new patterns for exploration.

## VISUALIZATION (V3)

In this section we will look a little more deeply into ways to explore the third eye as well as gain an understanding of other energy centers that can contribute to Kriya visualization practices.

## Third-Eye Gazing

We were introduced to the third eye and the practice of third-eye gazing in chapter 5 (see page 72) and in the Shambhavi Mudra exercise earlier in this chapter (see page 132).

Anatomically, this area runs from the spot between the eyebrows (the Bindu) and into the skull toward the upper nasal passages and surrounding areas of the brain.[2] But as noted, initially the exact anatomical location is not as important as the direction of your intention or field of focus. The third eye is seen by many spiritual traditions as the gateway to the inner sky and true Knowledge. In Kriya it is also utilized as the initial focus in concentrated attention. It is the third practice in Kriya, after posture and breath.

### Focused Awareness

The third eye gives the visual mind a place to focus its attention while also allowing you to become one with the sensations of your experience without judgment or rigidity. This is an example of one-pointed concentration, and this position of internal focus guides you to the seat of your inner vision. To begin with there may be nothing there, but with time shapes and colors may appear and as skill develops and combines with the synergy of posture and breath, a new level of experience opens up within the third eye allowing for true sight and Knowledge. If you experience visualization of a light or an object while third-eye gazing, allow yourself to stay with this experience. Focus your attention on the center of that light or object. This is the place where the gift of true sight begins to emerge.

> *The light of the body is the eye: if therefore thine eye be*
> *single, thy whole body shall be full of light.*
> MATTHEW 6:22

The path through the third eye is vast and goes well beyond the initial "light" that is often seen at first. With time, stillness, and focus one becomes aware of the deeper inner eye that takes over if one has developed the ability to stay mentally focused on the intial light and to travel through it. Cultivate your ability to connect with the light that shines within you. In Kriya it is not uncommon for this light to be experienced as an azure glow. Sometimes it also comes with a lighter white yellow center to it. It represents successful practice and was openly spoken about by Ganesh Baba. Although it does not happen for everyone as each experience with the divine has its own unique components.

One might also experience a magnet-like pull as one's attention is pulled to the third eye area, and one's inner vision appears clear as day. This often corresponds to a sense of deep pleasure and relaxation. One can even find that a soft and pleasant smile develops by itself. With time and grace other journeys within the inner sky will open themselves to you.

Although there is no absolute exact anatomical point where the third eye exists, one place where the inner sky can be recognized is in the area of the brain's frontal lobes. It is interesting to note that the general area of the frontal lobes is shown to be thicker in monks that have engaged in meditation over the years.[3]

## *Deepening the Practice of Third-Eye Gazing*

In this form of Kriya yoga we begin with our eyes closed. Many other forms of meditation begin with open eyes focused on a spot on the horizon. These variations of meditation also serve as forms of attention training and can be helpful for a beginning student. In addition, you may read about other areas on which to focus your attention such as deeper inside the skull or the tip of the nose. All these techniques provide some benefit, but the one technique that seems to help people move the quickest is focusing on the area between the eyebrows or just an inch or so higher or deeper than that. Remember to keep your eyebrows slightly raised in a relaxed fashion and, particularly for a beginner, to try "looking" at the third eye with a relaxed gazed from your peripheral vision as opposed to the center of your visual field. Once you are confident with your skill in this area try adjusting the focus of your inner field of vision and notice what else is there.

These are all ways to explore your own inner vision. The goal is to develop a relaxed but intent focus of awareness that becomes more refined as you gain experience.

As mentioned, the third eye has been associated with many anatomical components, including the forehead, the pituitary area, and the pineal gland area. The third eye in its deepest area has been referred to as Brahma's Cave and lies in a space close to the third ventricle (see figure 14.2 on page 223). All this will take time to explore. Although in the beginning, the best results occur by keeping the attention on the forehead just above the eyebrows, with time you may want to explore other various energetic centers.

## ≪ Cribriform Plate

One technique that can help develop a deep sense of calmness and engagement with the third eye is an awareness of the brain. To begin the exercise, bring the energy of the breath up through the nostrils and the cribriform plate (see figure 8.7) and into the brain above your eyes and into your frontal lobes. In other words, try pulling the breath from your nostrils into the forehead area through the sinus area just between and above your eyes. Feel the flow of the breath in your brain while at the same time feeling your lungs expand in all directions. The flow of a slow and even breath has its own effect on this area as our sense of smell is strongly related to survival. See if you can appreciate a deep calmness as the tiniest movement of air flows through your nasal cavity as you pull the breath into this area.

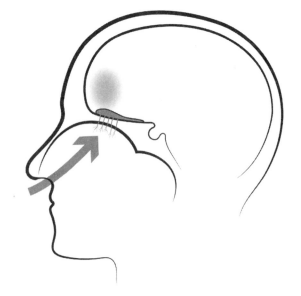

Figure 8.7. Cribriform plate. This is part of a tiny bone in our head that is tissue thin in places and is called the ethmoid bone. It is unique in that it has little holes in it that allow the olfactory nerve to send receptors through the skull and into our nasal cavity, which is how we are able to smell.

This is not a beginner breathing exercise, but once one has posture and basic pranayama down this can help in the development of Kriya visualization exercises. Play with this exercise and see what develops inside the forehead, on the forehead, and even in higher areas of the brain toward the vertex.

## Chakras

We have just spent time exploring the third eye also known as the ajna chakra. We will now take some time to explore the other chakras.

In yoga energy is referred to as prana and that prana is described as running through channels called nadis. There are said to be 72,000 nadis in the human body. From an energetic standpoint they are very similar to the Chinese medicine idea of meridians. The chakras are energy centers connected by these nadis. Neither of these systems have clear, one-to-one anatomical correspondences. The nadis are associated with a combination of nerves, blood vessels, and fascial planes.* The chakras are associated with the central nervous system, meaning the brain and the spinal cord, as well as the autonomic nervous system.

The seven main chakras represent different patterns of pranic energy that animate and give different characteristics to the various sections of the body (see figure 8.8 on page 146). Indian yoga and tantric teachings describe the chakras as beginning at the top of the skull and proceeding along the spine to the coccyx. From top to bottom, the chakras are as follows: the crown/fontanel chakra (top of the head), the third eye chakra, the cervical/throat chakra, the thoracic/heart chakra, the lumbar/abdominal chakra, the sacral/genital chakra, and the coccyx/root chakra.

Many individuals with and without a yoga practice experience energies in different chakras. Putting one's hand over one's heart when speaking about a heartfelt emotion or feeling a disruption in one's

---

*Fascia, which is a tissue very similar to the dura mater, is increasingly being recognized as an important mode of information transmission within the body and clearly contributes to the experience of kundalini, which is described in greater detail below.

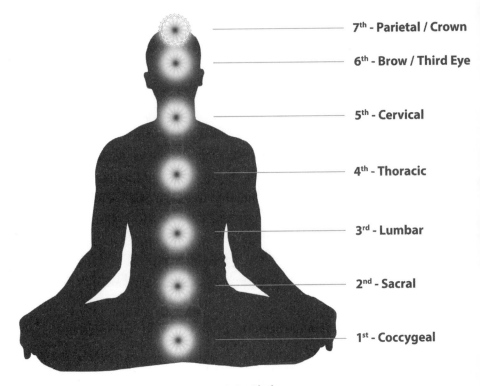

7th - Parietal / Crown

6th - Brow / Third Eye

5th - Cervical

4th - Thoracic

3rd - Lumbar

2nd - Sacral

1st - Coccygeal

Figure 8.8. Chakras.

abdomen when anxious are two examples. Kriya yoga as a whole helps one experience and ultimately manage these channels so that higher concentrations of pranic energy can occur in specific areas and movement of that energy can be encouraged in various ways.

The list below provides brief descriptions of each of the chakras along with their English and Sanskrit names. The elements of each chakra as they relate to yoga philosophy and Ayurvedic medicine are also noted. In general, the lower chakras are seen as being more connected with Nature and Creation and are associated with the five senses and the upper chakras are more associated with Spirit and Transcendence and are the areas that *experience* what the lower chakras *sense*.

7. **Crown Chakra (*Sahasrara*):** The crown chakra, also referred to as the "thousand petal lotus," includes the anterior and posterior fontanel areas on the head and the area between them referred to as the vertex. Both of these fontanels and the vertex area are involved energetically in the chakra system. The specific energy patterns within this chakra can vary based on the specific attentional focus at any given time. This is the highest chakra within the body, and it is right at the apex of our central nervous system. This chakra provides the most direct interface of the physical body with the subtle energetic fields described in the Cycle of Synthesis. This crown chakra is the last to open along the path when kundalini decides to rise from the root and make its presence known at the crown and beyond. Some lines of Kriya yoga recommend that beginning practitioners focus on the posterior fontanel area of this chakra, while others recommend they focus on the third eye. Clearly, both paths are useful and provide results. The Kriya yoga described in this book largely follows the form taught by Ganesh Baba, where the initial focus is on the third eye.

6. **Third Eye Chakra (*Ajna*):** This chakra is referred to as the third eye, or the gyral center, which is a term that seems to have been coined by Ganesh Baba and refers to the idea of a gyroscope that you can balance and ride inside the third eye. This chakra is the source of inner vision, intuition, and pure Knowledge, and it is from here that one transcends to the crown chakra.

5. **Cervical Chakra (*Visuddha*):** The cervical, or throat, chakra is not typically written about in great depth, but it is very important nonetheless. It is associated with the vacuum or ether element and corresponds with sound and the ears. Speech and the proper use of language, particularly when it is coming from the heart, is of the utmost importance and can carry great power. Untruths can lead to great distress therefore one must be mindful of what is spoken or thought. It is of note that this chakra is between the

third eye and the heart chakras, which are uniquely powerful in the path toward transcendence. The power of vibration is spoken about in other areas of this book, and it should be clear that our own instrument of creative vibration—our voice—comes from this chakra. Although there is great emphasis on hearing the inner sound, there is also great power in rhythmic vibrations stemming from humming or chanting in prayer. This is not an area to neglect and is one waiting for deeper exploration. Explore the joy of the vibration of sound and the power of the spoken word.

4. **Thoracic Chakra (*Anahata*):** The thoracic, or heart, chakra is one most people can relate to. It is associated with the air element and corresponds to touch and the lips. When developed the heart chakra provides the ability to engage in selfless love for all. This is the root from which compassion blooms. This area is of major importance in all self-regulatory techniques. Once one begins to work in this area, they are well on their way toward the greater awakening. Of course, heartache can be quite severe and lead to anger, jealousy, and depression, but one who is well-versed in the energy aspects of yoga and this chakra will be relatively unfazed in situations that might lead others to suffer. Someone well-versed in the practice of compassion and the use of the four Vs is much more able to transmute any negative emotional energy toward forgiveness.

3. **Lumbar Chakra (*Manipura*):** The lumbar chakra is associated with the fire element and digestion and corresponds to sight and the eyes. Reflecting on this chakra one has to wonder about the meaning behind the phrase "your eyes are bigger than your stomach." It is described as the center of pranic energy and is also associated with generosity and sustenance. Prana provides a source of energy for oneself and others, particularly when the engagement has to do with compassion. Anxiety, a challenging emotion, is often felt here. If the energy in this area is misused it can be a source of disruptive power.

**2. Sacral Chakra (*Svadhisthana*):** The sacral chakra is associated with the water element and taste and the tongue. It is also associated with sexuality and reproduction. When this chakra is out of balance it can lead to an obsessional focus and negative self-talk. With a greater awareness of the energetic body and meditative experiences, the active libidinous energy in the chakra begins to shift more toward the spiritual focus, which ultimately is a more sustainable source of bliss.

**1. Root Chakra (*Muladhara*):** The root, or coccyx, chakra is associated with the earth element and the sense of smell and therefore associated with the nose. Located near the tip of the coccyx, as its name implies, it is associated with the ground, so when it is active and engaged one feels stable and secure. Once one has a solid base everything else can begin to grow. Think of this chakra as your connection to the earth, which provides structure for sustainability, sustenance, shelter, and stability for your life. It is the area between the coccyx chakra and the sacral chakra, where kundalini energy sits and waits. Although one may not consider the coccyx chakra very important, it is in fact sitting at the base of the spine and is the tip of the sacrum, which holds the pelvis together and provides the basic structure from which the spine can rise straight up, on which our head rests, and in which the central nervous system resides. Given this, one could say that it is the most important chakra. And, as pointed out throughout this book, proper posture is key to practicing Kriya yoga, as once one carries their structure in anatomical proper alignment everything else can manifest on its own. The coccyx is at the base of that structure.

. . . . . . . . . . . . . . . . . . . . . . . . . . . . . . . . . . . . . . . .

## Kundalini Rising

What is often described as kundalini rising is experienced when an individual's feminine, creative energy that rests as potential energy at the base of the spine becomes activated and rises toward the crown chakra, where the masculine quality of awareness/transcendence comes in from above and the two meet. Kundalini can become activated either spontaneously or through a variety of techniques, such as Kriya yoga. As the creative energy rises, it meets and unites with the spiritual energy, leading to the beginning of the path toward Self-Realization. This is the underlying goal of yoga and tantra meditation. It is an energetic dance between the creative energies of Nature and the transcendent energies of Spirit that unite, allowing one to experience the Ultimate Universal Unity of nonduality.

With the practice of Kriya yoga one can experience a direct awakening of kundalini. The *sushumna* is the main channel of kundalini and is considered the primary nadi. The next two predominate nadis run on either side of the sushumna and are called *ida* and *pingala*. These two nadi correspond to the dual nature of the physical universe. The ida is on the left side and represents the feminine principle and the pingala is on the right side representing the masculine principle. It is the balancing of these flowing energy patterns that contributes to the release of kundalini.

Through the practice of Kriya yoga awareness of the sushumna and other nadis as well as the chakras will become more refined. While these energy channels and centers are directly related to the release of kundalini energy, kundalini does not necessarily first check in to see if the path ahead is clear for its rise. For this reason more direct exercises to raise kundalini do not occur at the beginning of the Kriya yoga practice. There are many reports of challenges with the rising of kundalini. But it was the experience of Ganesh Baba and myself that if one can first develop a solid practice of basic Kriya (V1 through V4), particularly posture (V1) and breath (V2), then the challenges with kundalini do not cause significant distress.

Kriya yoga focuses on posture and breath, which leads to increasing awareness of the intrapersonal and interpersonal behaviors associated with the yamas and niyamas. Once one begins to engage regularly in straight posture and straight breath, behavior begins to shift automatically. The addition of the third-eye focus exercises and heart-focused exercises such as loving-kindness (see page 228) move the practice along even faster. These activities coupled with mild to moderate physical exercise that emphasizes spinal flexibility and strength prepare the body and mind for the release of kundalini so that it, along with Self-Realization, is welcomed rather than feared.

· · · · · · · · · · · · · · · · · · · · · · · · · · · · · · · · · · · · · · · · · · · · · · · · · · · · · · · · ·

## *Micro-Modulations in Visualization (V3)*

There are many micro-modulations one can make to the third eye, or visualization. Initially there will likely be considerable adjustment as one explores the third eye and this will continue as one's journey progresses. Paramahansa Yogananda refers to the whole central nervous system as an area to explore and that, in fact, is the case. The third eye is the entryway to a vast inner universe that is beyond everyday conscious awareness. Once again, become sturdy and proficient in focusing on your mind's eye and as that focus becomes more routine, making very slight adjustments to your attentional focus will lead to the next opening. Your inner visual field is what micro-modulation helps fine tune. In other words, how broad or narrow the focus of your mind's eye is at any given time influences what is seen. The position and tension in the eyebrows also have an influence here. Micro-modulations in V3 can adjust one's acuity of the inner sky as well. This is a hard concept to understand at first but will become evident as one's practice develops. With time you may even be able to return to where you were in a previous meditation session.

## VIBRATIONALIZATION (V4)

As we have discussed vibration is an important part of Kriya yoga. Finding a few comfortable ways to include both vocal and silent vibrational focus in your practice is important. Below are a few specifics on how to begin this exploration.

## Sound, Vibration, and Mantra

The vocal repetition of a rhythmic mantra/sound, a spiritually charged phrase, or Om brings the breath deeper into the body while inviting awareness to expand to the outer reaches of oneself. Even the use of a soft background hum can be helpful in this regard. Most cultures that have a connection to the natural world have a practice of vocalizing meaningful phrases in rhythmic and resounding ways as do most spiritual groups. Sometimes people grow up with associations to various chants or hymns that hold deep meaning for them. Others receive a particular mantra from a guru, or spiritual teacher. These can sometimes be a great source to choose from if one wants a repetitive sound with a devotional focus. On occasion an individual experiences a spontaneous expression of a chant or mantra or is inspired to sing or hum. In such cases these vibrations are often very appropriate for the individual and following a prescribed culturally expected choice may not be as productive.

The bottom line here is to explore and find a vibrational phrase/ sound that resonates with your body, mind, and soul. It is good to briefly experiment with various expressions of this practice; however, it is very important to remember that choosing one variation and sticking with it is the way to truly progress. Stay with the core practices and play with your edges. The power of repetitive sound is vast and will grow in its significance as you embrace it. In Kriya practice we utilize Om as an aid to bring even greater awareness into the spinal column. This is primarily a silent practice, but you can explore using your voice as well. Your inner guide is there, and outer guides will present themselves as you need them. Go forward, go inward, and explore. This is only the beginning and the treasures in store are infinite and exponentially transforming.

## Micro-Modulations in Vibrationalization (V4)

The use of a repetitive internal vibration or sound can also be micromodulated and adjusted ever so slightly to see what effect it has on you and your nervous system. For example mantras can last for one cycle of inhalation and exhalation or can be used twice during the breath cycle, one on inhalation and one on exhalation. When repeating a sound or mantra, each repetition might have its own tone or note, creating a repetitive pattern, or might repeat a single tone. Another option is listening to and feeling the internal vibration of ocean breath as you hear the air flow through your throat and nasal passages on inhalation and exhalation.

## SPINAL AWARENESS OF ENERGY AND AN INTRODUCTION TO PLEXUS PLUCKING

Once one becomes accomplished in V1 through V4 more advanced techniques of spinal awareness are available. A basic introduction to plexus plucking (a term coined by Ganesh Baba) is included here. But as always, it is advisable to practice the more involved techniques under a more advanced practitioner if possible. Many have written and posted videos online about "rising kundalini," "Kriya pranayama," or "spinal breathing" in ways that are vague, confusing, or both. These techniques are very powerful and should not be engaged in lightly. With proper direction plexus plucking can help speed the process of kundalini rising in one who is well established in V1 through V4 practices. A goal of plexus plucking is to help activate kundalini by creating more focused energy in the chakras. Once the skill of plexus plucking is developed it can help clear the energy path of the sushumna of any blockages in someone who has mastered maintaining a bolt upright spine.

## ≫ Plexus Plucking

1. Beginning with an inhalation, feel the breath fill up your spinal column area with prana from the coccyx to the crown.
2. On the exhale feel the energy retreat back deep into the root chakra area. This practice should be slow and deliberate and be the focus of your attention.
3. Repeat Om or another mantra or sound with each inhale and exhale, or just on the inhale, maintaining a smooth, consistent, rhythmic flow of breath up and down the spine.

4. Practice remaining internally focused, listening to the vibrations within the body.

Just focusing on the spine itself is more than enough to move forward along the path or you can also bring in a focus on the chakras.

To do this, continue to use Om or another sound or mantra, maintain your focus up and down the spine but focus this awareness to move up and down chakra by chakra. Do not worry about where exactly the chakras are. That will come with time and is not necessary at this point. A general idea of their location is more than sufficient.

Another option is to focus on each chakra for a breath cycle breathing into each energy center. This will help you get more acquainted with the various energies at different levels.

You might also consider directing Om to the third eye as well as the fontanel and explore those experiences as exercises in themselves. (We will be doing this explicitly with the heart chakra later.) The goal here is to explore the spine and further refine your antenna.

In any of these variations, maintain your spine in a bolt upright position that is strong yet flexible, with a full breath that is relaxed and rhythmic as you actively concentrate on your spine.

---

Plexus plucking can be a very powerful exercise and should not be attempted until deep relaxation and contemplation occurs on a regular basis with proper breath and posture maintained. One should be adept at having all four Vs working in synchrony before plexus plucking is attempted.

## Micro-Modulations for Plexus Plucking

A micro-modulation for plexus plucking involves using the musical scale—do, re, mi, fa, so, la, ti—so that each chakra can have its own tone with the highest tone at the crown chakra and the lowest at the root chakra. In a way you are playing the chakras as a musical instrument. Although a little more complex, one can also recite the musical scale in typical fashion going up and in reverse on the way down.

This clearly requires a little more concentration and practice. Just as in vibrationalization, you could also focus on trying to hear the internal vibration, which often sounds like the buzz of insect wings, the inside of a conch shell, the hum of a small motor, or the sound you hear when you use your fingers to close your ears. With time, effort, experience, and subtle micro-adjustments, an increased understanding of these techniques will emerge and help you move forward. There are similar techniques that utilize Sanskrit words for each of the chakras. It was Ganesh Baba's opinion that the musical scale was just as effective as well as being easier for most westerners to use.

\* \* \*

In this chapter we have explored macro and subtle micro-modulations for V1 through V4 to experience and reflect on. We encourage a "slow and steady" practice that moves forward in moderation with appropriate respect and humility through a fine-tuned set of exercises. This fine-tuning of our antenna provides the reception for all the fields with which we will be interacting as we pursue the meditative process. As we breathe and reflect, visualize, and concentrate on these modulations, we gain increasing somatic awareness and insight about the subtle effects of our prana, our life force, and how we experience and feel the change throughout our core being. How we connect these macro and micro-modulations to breath will bring about even greater changes in our ability to concentrate. With each adjustment, allow time to reflect, visualize, and internalize the direction of prana in the body. The management of prana or life force energy is in the mastery of inhalation, retention, and exhalation. Remember this is a creative endeavor based on a sound time-honored structure that is strong and resilient. Play with it, love it, respect it, and it will do the same to you.

*Try to refrain from ingesting what others say about their meditative experiences and keep an inward focus of the senses. It is your own mind that does not allow you to meditate. Always return to the breath.*

## THE STILLPOINT

Awareness is cultivated through stillness, which is why meditation becomes the focus for achieving states of true Knowledge and Self-Realization. These techniques prepare the body and mind for the deep dive into the subtle (bio-psychic) and causal (intello-conscious) fields of energy where one mingles with the unconscious, conscious, and supra-conscious integrations. This process is deceptively simple but leads to infinitely creative and transcendent experiences. This is where the art and science of Kriya yoga come together and lead to spiritualization. It must be practiced, practiced, and practiced some more. Without practice little will happen. With practice all is possible and stillness reveals itself in ways that defy the imagination.

The goal of Kriya yoga is to feel the embodiment of breath in the space between each cell within one's body-mind and to find the balance between Spirit and Nature. This is the stillpoint. Another name for Lahiri Mahasaya's after-effect poise of Kriya. Stillness is discovered most easily though a loving relationship with the breath. It is the breath that controls the mind and the mind that controls the breath. Working with only the mind proves very challenging in the current world culture. Accessing our Spirit through our breath is a more immediate and tangible path toward Self-Realization. Spirit and body (Nature) recognize each other through the warm embrace of the breath. Stillness is the non-duality of the moment and beyond, the balance where time is no longer, the breathlessness moments of Ultimate Universal Unity where human experience of Knowledge of Cosmic Consciousness lies in wait.

Balance is at the root of all Kriya practices. It is only through ongoing refinement of balance that one's attention can fully turn inward and begin to see the light without the static. The static, whether it is physical stress or strain, emotional obsession, worry or anxiety, or hunger or fatigue pulls one's awareness away from engaging in the moment of stillness, of Self-Realization, keeping it just beyond one's grasp. When balance happens, one experiences the emergent properties of the Realization of the Self, which then merges with Cosmic Consciousness in all its glory.

Please remember, stillness is not out there; it is within you and around you. You do not need any particular teacher, technique, or relationship or a trip to some exotic location. All you need is to be straight in posture and breathe. Breathe the luscious air that surrounds you, do the work (kri) of the breath/Soul (ya), and join in the union of yoga.

## ❦ Combining Exercises into a Kriya Practice Session

Now that we have reviewed and tried the basic concepts and practice of posture and breath as well as visualization and sound, we will combine them all together in one session.

### Physical Movement

Before you begin, complete some form of limb limbering and some shoulder shuffling. As we have discussed this can be fairly brief, but it should be deliberate and systematic.

### Meditation Posture

Once you have completed your stretching and strengthening exercises, settle into a strong, relaxed base structure that will be able to support you for at least fifteen minutes or so. As you engage in Kriya, this posture will be subtly refined periodically to accommodate physical needs. That said, the less you need to adjust your posture during meditation, the deeper and more sustained your session will become. The goal of proper posture is for you to feel comfortable, firmly in control, relaxed yet upright, and attentive. Slowly move toward a deep sense of calmness and structural support in your bolt upright posture.

### First Breaths: R4

We begin with a full breath that includes the movement of our shoulders to help settle in to a solid posture. With the first few breaths shoulders go up and back on the inhalation and then down on the exhalation. Once we feel comfortable we move to deep and slow

R4 abdominal breath that slowly rises up from deepest parts of your pelvis, moves outward from side to side and front to back, and slowly expands your abdomen. Focus on and relish the deep grounding ability of breath to fill your foundation and connect you to the earth below. Remember to keep the abdominal muscles engaged to some degree. We are not looking for a greatly expanded abdomen.

As you continue your inhale you begin to feel the breath moving up into your thorax, your ribs expanding in all directions, and your sternum rising. Feel the widening of your chest as your ribs tug ever so gently on your sternum and spine as expansion occurs. Now as you continue the last bit of this inhalation you notice your shoulders rise slightly as you engage both shoulder blades to move toward the spine. This relaxed breath is then topped off at the edge of your throat. When you feel "full" you can swallow, or not, but do add a little pressure to your Adam's apple area/thyroid by tilting your chin down and hold/retain your breath for a second or two.

Then slowly, with your shoulders dropping down, let the exhale begin in a comfortable, relaxed fashion but with the sense that there is some resistance in the back of your throat. You may even notice a slight "ocean breath" sound, which is just fine. This type of full, reposed, rhythmic breath helps you settle into your physical base of support. At this point, continue more of the same with the breath getting ever so finer as the moments pass. This becomes the subtle breath of Kriya yoga. In time this is where your practice will likely start with little need for the next step. That said, in the beginning few months or years you can start immediately with jet breath if it feels right after one or more cycles of R4.

## Jet Breath

As established earlier, jet breath is typically done in quick succession of one breath after another or in sets of three that repeat themselves in a rhythmic fashion. You can experiment and see which rhythm suits you at the moment. Jet breath can be quite energizing and should not be practiced to excess. A dozen or so breaths should be more than sufficient to help you get on your way. Initially this type of rapid jet breathing may lead to a feeling of light-headedness even after just a few breaths. If that happens, you have done enough and can switch to the slow rhythmic breath previously described. It should be noted here that as your practice matures, the need for Jet Breath can become less and less as you are able to enter the domains easier due to efficiencies and expertise.

Begin jet breath with an initial focus on your navel with the idea that you will be forcing air out by contracting your abdominal muscles in rapid succession by visualizing your navel moving back toward your spine with a slightly upward trajectory of about 30 degrees. Engage the muscles with a rapid and fairly deep exhalation by contracting your abdominal wall in firm rhythmic fashion toward your spine as noted. This will produce a "jet" of air out your nostrils. Your mouth should be closed with your tongue resting gently behind your front teeth.

Some form of tissue or handkerchief is often helpful to have around for this exercise due to occasional nasal discharge. With each exhale you may also include lumbar mobilization (see figure 8.9), the slight forward tilting motion of your pelvis that exaggerates your lumbar curve. As you do this check your pelvic diaphragm/perineum and

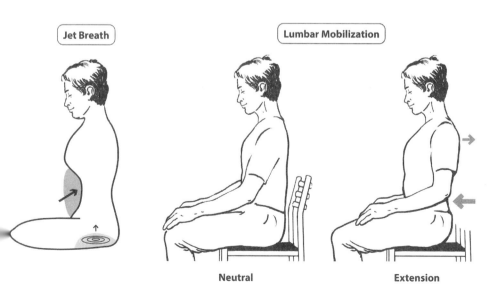

Figure 8.9. Jet breath and lumbar mobilization.

make sure it is engaged. In addition, remember to keep your erect posture, which includes keeping your shoulder blades back and bringing them closer together with the exhale. In fact you can also engage your shoulder girdle more vigorously with this exercise by using your arms as if they are wings (elbows bent with hands up toward the front of your body) and pulling your shoulder blades back as you exhale and gently bow your spine (extension) opening your chest as your elbows and shoulder blades move back.

Of course, this lumbar mobilization exercise is happening at the same time as the forced rapid jet breath is exhaled. This is all a bit complex at the beginning and sometimes feels completely backward and impossible to do. With a little practice, though, it will come together rather quickly. You may want to try practicing each aspect (jet breath, lumbar mobilization, and wings/shoulder shuffling) separately and then combine them together. Once you get the hang of it, this technique can be used at any time to refocus and energize your meditation if you have become distracted or have lost focus and want to reengage and reenter the deeper and slower R4. Remember this is a practice not to overdo. In small bursts it is without exception extremely powerful and effective.

## Return to R4

Once the jet breath portion is complete, you will naturally shift back into an R4 breath, which is often very deep initially but will become less so with time (see page 100 for a review of R4). As your breath shifts, return your attention to your posture for a moment. When shifting your breathing pattern, it's sometimes helpful to consciously readjust your posture. With the next inhalation, bring your shoulders up toward your ears, pause, and then move your shoulders back and down as you exhale. Feel your shoulders relax and let go. Repeat this until you feel your shoulders have had sufficient movement to keep them flexible and then continue with R4 breath without any shoulder movement beyond that which comes naturally.

The is a time to work with the refinement of relaxed, reposed, rhythmic respiration (R4) by deeply exploring the four aspects of inhalation, retention with full breath, exhalation, and retention with empty lungs. The goal over time is to develop a subtle, nurturing breath that is a source of calmness and joy. The breath itself can become extremely deep and delectably delicious allowing you to feel the intoxicating nectar of the infinite—the Kriya breath. This dance begins with inhalation, deepens with retention, is explored through exhalation, and is repeated with the next breath. This is the time in a Kriya session to deepen the exploration through ocean breath.

## Ocean Breath with Neck Lock (Jalandhara Bandha)

Now add ocean breath, which occurs when you focus your attention on the neck bandha. This further refines the breath process as we are continuing R4 at the same time. In order to engage this bandha, make sure your posture is straight then slowly elongate your spine further as you tilt your head forward from the C7 vertebra (the one that sticks out the most on the back of your neck). As you do this, feel the cervical part of your spine lengthen as the neck stays straight but its natural curve slightly flattens and lengthens as your head moves forward. As you breathe, the upper part of the chest will rise and move toward your chin. At the same time you can also engage the muscles in your throat and constrict them slightly to provide some resistance to the air as it passes through your oropharynx. This technique helps slow the breath down, provides some physical resistance to the breath, extends the spine to help with energetic flow, and provides some additional vibration in the back of the throat and nasopharynx, which is in close proximity to the brainstem/medulla oblongata, the seat of the autonomic nervous system and has profound influence on our awareness and state of consciousness. The goal is to integrate ocean breath with R4 of Kriya.

Once this combination of ocean breath with R4 is mastered to some degree you can explore the edges and try some different rate and volume ratios for the four parts of the breath as previously discussed (see pages 102–3). When exploring retention first focus on retention with inhalation. The goal is deep and rhythmic patterns that move to a subtle almost delicate flow. Retention adds a lot to this process. Ultimately, it will probably be the simplest patterns that will provide the deepest, long-lasting at the beginning. It is the subtle relationship between inhalation, retention, and exhalation that is the essential ingredient in Kriya breathwork.

## Vacuum Breath, or Modified Uddiyana Bandha

Whether or not you find the retention on inhalation aspect of the breath challenging, it is useful to play with vacuum breath during R4 (retention on exhalation). When you are ready, exhale completely using your abdominal muscles to push all the air out and then practice retention of the breath on exhalation until you feel the need to proceed with an inhale. Do not retain the breath to the point that you will be gasping for breath. When you inhale, do it *passively*. Relax and let go of your abdominal muscles and allow the pressure gradient that was set up with the forced exhale to quickly fill your lungs with a big swishing sound as the air enters and the pressure equalizes. An additional element to this exercise is to work your abdominal muscles after the exhalation and during the retention by sucking in your abdomen as if you are trying to take a breath but do not let any air enter. Try to do this in a rhythmic fashion while you maintain your retention. This provides additional training in breath awareness while at the same time toning your abdominal muscles and massaging your abdominal organs. The goal with time is to integrate a mild form of this on occasion at the end of exhalation during R4. This is a fun, stimulating, and centering practice. It is helpful to do this by itself at times or to return to it when your meditation has stalled during a session for whatever reason.

You are now practicing Kriya pranayama. Feel into each element of the breath techniques and explore the relationship between them and your experience within. The goal here is to increase your respiratory fitness and control so that the world of breath modulation can be deeply explored. Ultimately with practice and perseverance these breath ratios will have little to no relevance as the right flow for the moment will always be present within your meditation. These exercises are a means to an end. You must master enough of the breath to be able to play the game. In order to get there one needs to build a reservoir of prana and know how to fill it, maintain it, and utilize it. Kriya breath is poetry in motion. Play with it. Explore it. It will lead you down the royal path. Remember, it is all in the breath.

## Adding Visualization (V3) and Vibrationalization (V4)

Once you find that you can sit straight (V1) and engage in jet breath to the point where you move into deep R4 with retention without much stress or strain (V2), you can begin to move to the next level of integration, visualization (V3). Once that is established add vibrationalization (V4). It is fine to explore aspects V1 through V4 at random at the beginning but mastering them in order will provide the fastest progress. Once you feel you have a good handle on one practice add the next. When all V1 through V4 practices happen in a synchrony without much thought or effort, Kriya yoga meditation can take hold.

A good place to start with V3 is with the previously described exercise of pulling breath through the nasal passage up into the third eye area. Kriya is an experiential path. Engage in the exercise and feel it. Get acquainted with this area of your forehead and forebrain. A regular, reposed, rhythmic breath that is smooth and subtle will go a long way in providing the foundation for V3 to begin to establish itself.

Once you feel some sense of confidence with V3 move forward and add V4. You can start with V4 in a myriad of ways. There is no right or wrong here. If you have a repetitive sound/mantra practice you can just add it here. For people who are first exploring repetitive sound in the mind's ear a gently rhythmic pattern of Om in the background is a good place to start. Keep it simple with one Om for both the inhale and exhale or one on the inhale and another on the exhale. The goal again is to have a nice smooth cadence to this inner voice. Another good introductory technique to try once V3 is established is to bring the Om to the third eye area. In this way you are bringing the mind's eye and the mind's ear together so to speak in the third eye area. This practice can quickly bring a new depth to your meditation.

## Encouragement toward Meditation

At this point you have gone through a number of different breathing exercises and it is time to practice and play. Remember that while the basics of straight back and R4 breath should always be maintained, the rest is all relative and depends on your desire, energy, physical fitness, and mental fortitude at any given time. Please remember that this is not a contest. It is a slow careful investigation of consciousness from within. Avoid trying to push your practice too quickly. Start with five minutes twice daily and move up to fifteen minutes twice daily if you can do so comfortably.

## Practice, Practice, Practice

The true secret to successful Kriya yoga meditation is simply this: PRACTICE. While all serious students receive this instruction, many do not give it the respect it deserves. If you practice regularly, even in small amounts, your life will change in ways that are hard to imagine.

---

PART III

# THE SCIENTIFIC
# EFFECTS OF
# KRIYA YOGA

# 9

# Wellness, Stress, Psychology, and Kriya Yoga

*Stillness of breath equals stillness of mind.*

Today, the general population throughout the world suffers significantly from various types of depression and anxiety. Some of this is caused by stress, some by the environment, some by various forms of trauma/abuse, and some by the atrocities of war. This results in interpersonal difficulties, poor health, violence, and further trauma.

Modern civilization provides little in the way of guidance for working with stress so that it does not become overwhelming. Although many people exercise and are aware of meditation and yoga benefits, more can be done to influence young people early in their lives so they understand how to balance stress in daily life.

In the past, societies worked more actively to dissipate chronic stress through regular movement like dance, competition, play, and physical endurance exercises. They also prepared people for the need to fight a threat, and taught them how use aggression appropriately. These are all ways the body self-regulates stress hormones and responses to return to baseline. Recreational activities burn up stress hormones, or catecholamines, such as epinephrine (adrenaline) and norepinephrine and provide benefits mostly by focusing on the sympathetic part of the autonomic nervous system, which is what is activated in the well-known flight-or-fight response. Meditation, however, focuses on intentionally activating the parasympathetic nervous system, which is a branch of the autonomic nervous system as previously discussed. This system allows for a restorative physiological process to occur.*

We must consider the term *stress* and how it has been taken out of context and confused with overuse. It now represents everything from worry to panic, is credited for a multitude of physical ailments, and can be an instigator in many mental wellness concerns. Stress has gotten a bad reputation, but it is actually multidimensional and like emotions, it has both positive and negative aspects.

For example, there are multiple stressors going on in your body at this moment. On a microscopic scale, there are millions of exchanges occurring within each cell. Every time a neuron fires anywhere in your body, electrical-chemical gradients maintained by your neurons provide transmission signals that allow your brain to make sense of the input. This becomes experience, and this electrical gradient is a form of stress across the neuron's cell membrane. Without it the nervous system would not function properly. Nerves actively use this energy to activate ions with electrical charge, thereby changing the concentration gradient across the membrane of the neuron. When a neuron fires, it is this relative balance of electrical charge that when given the opportunity, moves toward equilibrium and decreases the stress on the cell caused by unequal charges inside and outside of a cell. This is an example of how the intelligence of the body is calibrated to use certain stresses to its advantage and how the brain uses stress to move a signal from one part to another. This is a positive form of stress in that there is a continuous counterbalancing at play.

---

*Dr. Herbert Benson, a Harvard cardiologist, initially not interested in researching meditative effects, coined the term "relaxation response" after research proved that transcendental meditation was effective as a simple way to induce parasympathetic tone and return the body to pre-stress levels.

On the other hand, a neuron can be sensitized to fire when there is no need to, such as during a panic attack. This is an example of a hyperexcitable neuron or group of neurons that get stimulated when they should be at rest. Such a response can be triggered by reexperiencing an extraneous stimulus that occurred at an earlier time of chronic stress or trauma. An example of this would be hearing a certain song that was playing when one received the news that a loved one had passed away. Hearing the song at a later time could activate the sadness and loss again out of the blue. This is also what happens in PTSD.

Even breathing causes stress on the system. Oxygen attaches to the hemoglobin molecule and depending on the concentration gradients of oxygen and other factors there is either attachment or release of the oxygen molecule. This is another example of the stress of a concentration gradient moving across the thin membranes in one's lung, which allows for the exchange of oxygen from the air to the blood. The physical act of breathing expands our chest and puts stress on our ribs to move in one direction and then another. On inspiration, our diaphragm incurs stress as it contracts. And of course, our heart is one of the easiest examples of stress to understand. Each heartbeat is an intense contraction of muscle that pushes blood into the pressurized arterial system. Too little stress would impair the arteries' function as they would not have the blood pressure to sustain proper flow, which can lead to passing out, and too much stress could cause a multitude of cardiovascular difficulties.

The body endures many daily stressors as well, including environmental toxins, psychoemotional stress, and poor diet, and these can cause an imbalance in the body, which can have disruptive effects and lead to disease in the mind and body. Too much stress is an obvious negative, but so is too little stress that prevents the system from performing properly.

Hans Selye was an innovative Canadian endocrinologist who, in the 1950s, coined the term "general adaptation syndrome," which described how stress can progress if not checked. The first stage is an initial alarm. Then there is a stage of resistance, at which point there is an attempt to adapt to the stressors. If resistance is not possible, then a state of exhaustion or burnout can ensue. As burnout approaches there is a decrease in personal health and well-being, poor relations with others, substance abuse, aggressive behavior, and ultimately emotional, physical, intellectual, and spiritual exhaustion. This type of stress leads to "disorders of arousal," which in turn lead to addictions, anxiety issues such as PTSD, panic, mood disorders, phobias, tendencies to dissociate, aggravated seizures, and distorted perceptions, as well as a number of physical disorders including cardiovascular complications, pain, and gastrointestinal and reproductive issues.

There are other much more insidious forms of stress that have become more present in recent human existence. If a person's living situation is not particularly safe, and their nervous system is forced to remain on high alert, it is increasingly difficult to rebalance. Chronic stress occurs over a period of time and inhibits the individual's ability to recover from what may have been minor stressors. Severe stress that becomes chronic leads to dysregulation of multiple physiological systems. As shown, human life would not be possible without some level of stress; the key is how we manage it and learn to cope with it, and how we grow to become more resilient as a community so we can assist each other.

## KRIYA YOGA, PSYCHOLOGY, AND THE PURSUIT OF WELLNESS

In medicine today the idea of disease prevention is well entrenched as medicine remains steeped in a disease model. Unfortunately, "prevention" often means the early detection of a disease process that has already begun. This idea is not the same as wellness. To that end we ask, what does it mean to be healthy, to have wellness? It is not merely the absence of disease but rather a continual striving for balance biologically, psychologically, and spiritually on a wellness spectrum (see figure 9.1 on page 170). To live a life with optimal health is a different

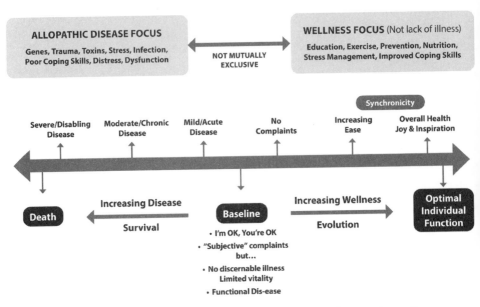

Figure 9.1. Wellness spectrum. This diagram is an extrapolation of a wellness continuum first outlined by John Travis, M.D., an Australian physician in 1972.

concept altogether, and it is the backbone of yoga and the goal of all aspects of the human experience.

Reversing the effects of toxic stress is important to our progress both as individuals and as a society. And there are many specific exercises to help retrain and rejuvenate the autonomic nervous system, mitigating the negative effects of toxic stressors. The consistent practice of health maintenance goes a long way to improving resilience so that chronic stressors and traumas have less of an effect on the overall system. The most basic of these include consistent and regular sleep, exercise, practice of self-regulatory techniques, a supportive social environment, and eating whole, minimally processed food.

In addition, paying attention to one's thoughts and belief systems during these times is very important, as our thoughts are very powerful. What is your mindset? There is a saying "you are what you eat" but just as appropriate is "you are what you think." The mind is very capable of creating our reality, and negative thought patterns are not something to take lightly. Becoming aware of negative thoughts and redirecting them to rewire old associations is something to aspire to. Faith or religious practices can support this endeavor, and techniques such as focusing on lines from prayers or positive phrases and affirmations can be very helpful as well, particularly when combined in a structured way with proper posture and breath.

There is a wealth of literature written on the physical, psychological, and spiritual benefits of practicing yoga. In contemporary Western research, medicine, psychiatry, and psychology have all shown the benefits associated with meditative and physical yoga practices for a wide variety of diseases and disorders. Meditative and self-regulatory techniques have been demonstrated to increase resilience and improve physical and psychological symptoms already present in existing conditions such as asthma, diabetes, hypertension, and infertility.

Early research in yoga-based meditation techniques was conducted by Herbert Benson, M.D., a Harvard cardiologist. He initially demonstrated the benefits of transcendental meditation on hypertension and went on to conduct many more studies. His first study, "A Wakeful Hypometabolic Physiologic State," was published in 1971 in the *American Journal of Physiology* with Robert Keith Wallace, Ph.D., and other studies quickly followed. Shortly thereafter research found that the practice of mindfulness techniques, as popularized by Jon Kabat-Zinn, Ph.D. in a mindfulness-related study in 1982, benefitted a variety of stress-related medical difficulties. In recent years specific forms of Kriya yoga such as Sudarshan Kriya, a proprietary meditation technique,[1] have been identified in the psychiatric literature as techniques that can help depression and obsessive-compulsive disorder. It is difficult to find any physical or psychological element that is not exacerbated by stress. Likewise, it is difficult to find any self-regulatory technique, utilized regularly, that does not decrease the negative aspects of stress in any individual.

Yoga has within its core philosophy an evolutionary-focused psychology. It is like many early holistic systems that were more integrated with Nature and emphasized the seamless connection between body, mind, and spirit. The practice of yoga is one that moves toward psychospiritual integration by working from the bottom up and from the top down at the same time. The physical aspect of yoga focuses on proper alignment and posture to support the foundation for a controlled connection with the Infinite through the breath-focused self-regulatory practice of pranayama, which settles the mind and helps regulate our emotions. The final integration in yoga comes when Spirit enters and connects with Nature, meaning when one is deeply grounded while at the same time in connection with the Infinite often experienced as the "awakening of kundalini," as described in the last chapter. As this occurs, one's self becomes aware of a deeper Knowledge, the beginnings of Self-Realization. This Self-Realization, or the experience of the infinite Self to put it another way, changes one's perspective of the human experience of the individual self from that point forward.

The contemporary development of somatic psychology has recognized yoga's evolutionary focus and is changing the Western idea of the body-mind split. This is being done with the age old practice of somatic embodiment, which promotes reintegrating the body, mind, and soul to optimize human function, transcend trauma, and allow an individual to find wholeness again.

Human beings possess an innate intelligence in every aspect of who they are. True healing simply removes obstacles and provides support so that the innate intelligence within can do its work toward integration. Current modern Western psychological theories focus primarily on illness treatment as opposed to optimal development. There were early individuals that studied the mind and realized there was more to healing it than treating hysteria. William James, Carl Jung, Abraham Maslow, Erik Erikson, and Elmer E. and Alyce M. Green represent only a handful of all the psychiatrists and psychologists to venture down that path.

Western psychological theories have been beneficial in helping us understand various levels of human development, particularly child development from an emotional and cognitive point of view. We now have greater comprehension of trauma and the ego and how the disconnect can clearly get in the way of our humanity. Unfortunately, societies have become increasingly isolated from Mother Nature and connections with the natural world have been lost.

Most native cultures had a deep understanding of their connectedness with Nature, and it informed their spiritual practice and understanding of their connection with powers greater than themselves. Many people turn to these cultures and their practices for guidance on how to incorporate natural wisdom once again in their busy lives. One of these practices is, of course, Kriya yoga. It is through the simple and regular practice of Kriya's self-regulatory techniques that psychospiritual integration can occur and help one move along an evolutionary path and influence civilization with more compassion and awareness. These techniques can markedly improve one's resilience and resistance to stressors and improve one's general health, wellness, and sense of joy and contentment in daily life. Although all self-regulatory techniques contribute to moving one in this general direction, Kriya yoga is of particular interest in that it can accelerate the process of experiencing a deep sense of inner contentment early on in one's practice.

Gaining understanding of and insight into oneself is the important part of yoga and psychotherapy, and in yoga it includes the intra-, inter- and transpersonal aspects of one's being. Psychology in yoga further acknowledges the connection between the mind and body and that the body must be part of the movement toward psychological and spiritual health and development. It is often one's "ego" that interferes with this by being overinflated, grandiose, and self-important or anxious, self-deprecating, and negativistic. But by including the body through posture and breathwork, the path to getting past the ego can be greatly accelerated. It is often said that there is a transcendence of the individual ego that is experienced by those moving along the spiritual path.

This is in fact what is supported by the integration of body and mind through the practice of yoga.

Ultimately the most significant difference with Western psychology suggested above is that in yoga the "mind" is not seen as the ultimate reality in itself but merely a filter/sensory organ through which one experiences a greater reality. The ego/self is the force that ties one to the mind and the limited interpretation of the ultimate reality that is the experience of greater Consciousness itself. It is through meditation that Consciousness can be experienced and can lead to new insights regarding one's mind/self and the ultimate experience of Nature and Spirit. It is through breath that one mediates the mind.

A well-known analogy used in contemplative traditions is that the mind is like the ocean and the waves. The ocean is the Self, the universal mind so to speak, and the waves are one's individual thoughts. Imagine swimming in the ocean or a large lake. On a stormy day (one filled with restless thoughts or anxiety), it is very busy at the surface with many waves and even wind. But go below the surface and the quiet begins. The deeper you, go the quieter it becomes. This is what meditation is all about. Meditative techniques such as Kriya yoga teach us to go below to the stillpoint where the motion of restless thoughts, or waves, have no real influence.

In general, the psychology of yoga sees the practice of yoga as a technique that "removes obstacles" and helps move one toward wellness as defined in the broadest sense. Yoga by itself can provide the needed integration that Western psychotherapy often struggles to find. The focus of yoga psychology is on the ongoing development of each human being as well as health and joy. The ultimate goal is the integration of the individual self with the larger Self by transcending the ego. The unconscious is accepted and in fact is seen as broad and universal as described by Carl Jung in his idea of the collective unconscious. Spirituality, or a space where daily religious and spiritual practices are supported, is also seen as necessary to integrate psychological wholeness.

## SELF-REGULATION IN A DISTRACTED WORLD

The challenge of maintaining a regular practice of self-regulatory techniques in the current time is that our attention is pulled on every moment by a variety of distractions. Cell phones, computers, and social media interrupt our daily lives with constant regularity. We are inundated with electronically delivered stimulus and conflicting data round-the-clock. We sleep next to electronic devices and spend much of our waking hours obsessively checking these same devices for the next scandal, news story, or bit of advice. Some meditation masters have called these electronic screens the "devil." Much of our awareness is devoured by the promise of the next electronic titillation. Studies are beginning to show a correlation between the way our brains seek pleasure and how these screens provide stimulation. We are, it seems, becoming addicted to our devices.

Where we direct our attention, life follows. Attention is one of the most beautiful gifts we can give, and it has been vacuumed up into a "virtual" void. We live in a vast expanse of glorious abundance. Nature surrounds us even in a dense metropolis, and this living planet is ever-ready to provide us with its bounty, yet our gaze and attention are directed toward nonliving, nonessential information that while prolific is far from life promoting.

We might begin to contemplate how the following are all related: the balance in nature's rhythms, the balance in self-regulation, the relationship or lack thereof between our attention and the rapidly changing planet, our level of health or disease, and trauma, violence, and the patterns that ensue and play out in nature. Despite the awareness of possible environmental catastrophe or cost to human lives, the West has not proved capable of restraining its appetite for consumables and technology. Progress since the dawn of the industrial age has had its risks, and these became starkly clear by the 1960s with the planning of the first Earth Day and Rachel Carson's book, *Silent Spring*, followed in the 1970s by Francis Moore Lappé's *Diet for a Small Planet*, all of which began to bring attention to some of the environmental tragedies that were unfolding around the globe.

The shift toward the degradation of resources is not unknown, but the sheer willingness of humans to destroy the planet in the race for corporate profit should be a deep shock to us all. What was a reasonably balanced ecological system has, in a mere few hundred years, turned into a massive reorganization of resources from which we will not recover in many lifetimes. This is not to say that the Earth is ending, as Mother Nature is an enduring and ever-renewing force. But for her to sustain humans, plants, and animals, she must have a modicum of support from and a balanced relationship with humans as well as some defense against their seemingly insatiable appetite for consumption.

What has yet to be fully realized is that our preparation for the future is not about the storage of food or water, toiletries, gold, or ammunition but an internal shift toward compassion, self-regulation, and balanced humility. No amount of external regulations, laws, or treaties will suffice. Our time has come to choose. It is now time for humans to change from within—from the heart. The heart, the spirit, and human beings' unique and innate intelligence must come together in an integrated fashion so that we can move forward as one to make appropriate changes for all of us. The individual focus of Western countries will become a thing of the past, as individuals cannot survive alone. We will need to ascend in our collective consciousness and be able to shine a light on the moments ahead.

We often overlook the power of our daily routine and the importance of self-regulatory practices. Being aware of oneself is the single most powerful act one can perform for the planet. Rather than becoming lost in the mire of what we have done wrong or how much pain we have endured at the hands of someone else, we can use each day to reset our internal network and reclaim the joy and the gift of our personal choices. But to do so, we must come into alignment with morals, ethics, and the cycles of nature, taking personal responsibility for our actions and their consequences, even if those actions were indirectly impactful.

If we do not take responsibility because we believe the resulting effects are still years away, that does not mean we are any less accountable for the actions, which may have a lasting and far-reaching impact on all of humanity.

The Iroquois nation had a constitution called the Great Binding Law. History suggests that this small democracy of six Native American tribes came together to live under a common law. One particular point made in the constitution was that governance would focus on the future: "Look and listen for the welfare of the whole people and have always in view not only the present but also the coming generations, even those whose faces are yet beneath the surface of the ground—the unborn of the future Nation."[2]

There is certainly enough time in everybody's day to devote fifteen minutes to the practice of Kriya yoga, or some other self-regulatory technique, which in itself will yield many benefits, but it must be a conscious choice. Since this would mean fifteen fewer minutes of screen time, do you think you can make and manage that change?

Moving away from technological distractions will help to improve mental wellness. While social connectedness is what holds our civilization together, social consciousness relies on each individual to be able to contribute in a way that moves society forward. Should we succeed as a species in moving from a fear-based survival to a compassionate, loving, and connected life, the entire planet will feel its benefits. This is not to say the practicing Kriya yoga will reverse global warming, negate nuclear waste, remove plastic from the oceans, clean up toxic dumps, or return extinct species to the planet. Practicing yoga will, however, influence the civilization to take more conscious action toward these endeavors. Mindful awareness makes recognition of the Divine Nature of all sentient beings more possible.

May we all acknowledge the challenge of our times and begin to look around and see when and where we can help. A great turning point is now upon us, and those with deep wells of compassion will be in great need and hopefully it will be those who will be asked to lead.

# 10

# Kriya Yoga, the Autonomic Nervous System, and the Development of Resiliency

---

*Practice, practice, practice.*

---

When we speak of intelligence, it's the brain that we often imagine first. A more complete truth, however, is that the entire body is perceiving its environment at all times, making adjustments to better harmonize with what is occurring and continually learning how to respond. The body is inherently intelligent in its perceptions of patterns and possesses an inherent awareness independent of the cognitive aspect of our brain. This forms the basis of theory in somatic psychology, a rediscovered ancient field of study that is growing more popular.

Just as our brain operates to catalog memories, experiences, or overwhelming/traumatic events, our bodies hold memories that interface with daily life and contribute to our overall perceptions. We are in a sense experiencing a self-perpetuating mind/body feedback loop that continues to build upon previous data to navigate through an ever-shifting landscape.

This form of intelligence cannot simply be explained as electrochemical or neurotransmitter communication. Subatomic particles, molecules, and atoms, too, have their own innate intelligence. They can recognize each electric charge, potential, and shape and intermingle in order to change their function and create a new dynamic. One might see this as just a series of three-dimensional molecules being pushed and pulled by positive and negative charges, but it is the Intelligence of Nature that drives that mechanism of an electric charge to develop in the first place. We continue to try to slice and dice intelligence in an attempt to form a distinct understanding of it, but central to it all we must recognize Nature as having its own innate Intelligence. We live together on an intelligent planet with every ecosystem managing its own checks and balances. The body is no different. Each of its systems is alive and continues to adapt in response to stresses or strains in order to develop, grow, and evolve. Through this we see the Intelligence of Nature, whose creativity has no end.

## AUTONOMIC NERVOUS SYSTEM AND THE POLYVAGAL THEORY

Our bodies contain a wonderfully complex and integrated central nervous system that ultimately defines how we experience ourselves and how others experience us. We may think of some of our abilities such as reaching for a cup of water as fairly rudimentary when in fact we still cannot quite get robots to do it with the same ease, finesse, and spontaneity that a human can.

This central nervous system consists of the brain and spinal cord, the autonomic nervous system, and a peripheral nervous system with a somatic component, which controls the movement of muscles. The autonomic nervous system has two branches—the sympathetic nervous system and the parasympathetic nervous system (see figure 10.1 on page 180)—and does all its work without much direction from our conscious thoughts. It is the interaction of the central nervous system with the autonomic nervous system, the parasympathetic nervous system in particular, that we are most concerned with in this discussion.

The autonomic nervous system controls the bodily functions that we do not have to think about, such as blood pressure, digestion, heartbeat, and breathing, as well as many other life-sustaining functions. With an increase in sympathetic tone we experience arousal, anxiety, fear, and muscle contraction, breathing becomes rapid and the heart races. In a parasympathetic response the opposite occurs: the gastrointestinal tract receives and digests food, heart rate slows, blood pressure is lowered, and energy is conserved. It is the part of our nervous systems that helps replenish and restore.

Historically, the sympathetic nervous system was thought to be the branch of the autonomic nervous system that was primarily in charge, so to speak. It was regarded as the engine that powered everything up or down in order to relax and allow the parasympathetic nervous system to monitor restoration, repair, and reproduction. What we are beginning to better understand is that each branch has a significant role to play

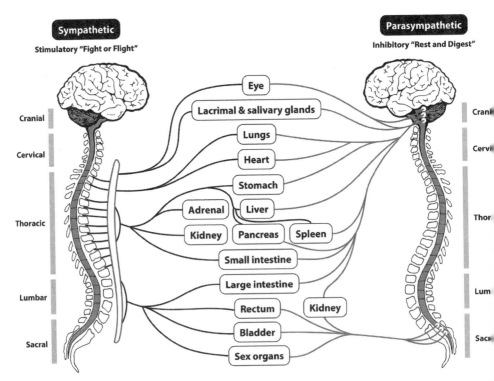

Figure 10.1. Autonomic nervous system.

and a responsibility to help manage and monitor the role of the other. Our ability to rev up the sympathetic nervous system is well developed, but we are lacking in techniques to strengthen and empower the parasympathetic nervous system. It is the latter that is capable of activating the vagal nerve so that it in turn can influence the entire system and our sense of well-being as well as prevent disease.

In his early work with the autonomic nervous system, physiologist Stephen Porges, Ph.D., refers to what he calls a "the vagal brake," which describes the parasympathetic nervous system and vagus nerve's strong governing effect on the sympathetic nervous system. In fact, one can think of the parasympathetic nervous system, which includes the vagus nerve, as providing a braking effect on the sympathetic nervous system, which would otherwise run amok. This is an important piece to understand from the standpoint of managing stress and anxiety.

The vagus nerve is an integral link between the heart, lungs, and digestive tract. Its name means "to wander" and it does wander through the body innervating and influencing the function of most internal organs. One could say that the vagus nerve is the one nerve most intimately and acutely impacted by negative stress as it is the centerpiece of the parasympathetic nervous system. It interfaces with the parasympathetic control of these organs and serves to communicate sensory information to the brain from all the internal organs. For example, the heart has its own internal beat, but it relies on the vagus nerve to sync it to the needs of the body. The heartbeat is significantly influenced by both the sympathetic and parasympathetic branches of the autonomic nervous system.

The important point here is the beat-to-beat variability, called "heart rate variability," that occurs in one's heart rate. Heart rate variability measures the relationship between the sympathetic and parasympathetic nervous system and is particularly sensitive to the influence of the vagal nerve. You may have actually observed heart rate variability and not realized it. If you visited someone in the hospital, and their heart rate was being monitored, there would have been a display showing the heart rate vary from 60, to 75, to 92, and so on, every second or so (see figure 10.2). If you felt the individual's pulse at that point in time, however, you would not have noticed a difference, as our touch is not sensitive enough to pick up the slight variations.

It was heart rate variability that formed the foundation for Dr. Porges's work. It can be seen in action with respiratory sinus arrhythmia, which refers to the body's ability to sense the difference between an inhalation and an exhalation and automatically adjust the heart rate to be faster when oxygen is coming in and slower when carbon dioxide is being expelled. Heart rate variability is considered a measure of health and resiliency. It is a reflection of one's adaptive physiology and ability to respond to stressors and return to a relaxed state. The greater one's heart rate variability, the greater one's ability to adapt to change. Kriya yoga and other pranayama techniques have taken advantage of this for thousands of years. Science is now catching up. Western society puts little to no emphasis on learning about self-regulatory practices that contribute to improving vagal tone. In fact, most of what is taught in school has to do with doings things faster, bigger, and better than the competition. The vagus nerve is more about cooperation than competition. In fact what we need is for kindergarten to teach self-regulatory skills so that children can learn at a young age to increase their vagal tone and govern their sympathetic nervous system, avoiding some of the overwhelming negative

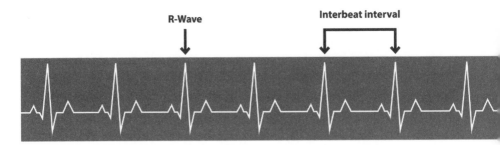

Figure 10.2. Heart rate variability. The electrocardiogram is showing the electrical impulse of a heartbeat as it travels through the muscle and electrical system of the heart.

effects stress has on their physical, psychological, and spiritual health and well-being.

I first wrote about Dr. Porges's work in a chapter on self-regulatory techniques in the late 1990s.[1] I chose his work to demonstrate what I thought at the time would be the most relevant active research in the mental health field in the coming decades. The chapter was published in 2000 and since that time, Dr. Porges's work continues to receive increasing amounts of attention in the mental health community.

Given my background in Kriya yoga. I was always deeply interested in the subcortical parts of the brain, as they clearly could have a mind of their own. Dr. Porges's work has developed as the *polyvagal theory,* a term coined by him. This is a relatively new theory that attempts to describe the vagus nerve's profound influence on a human's ability to feel safe and connect with others; in other words, their ability to relate socially. His theory has been enriched by his wife, C. Sue Carter, Ph.D. whose research has focused on oxytocin, love, and social bonds.

In the polyvagal theory, Dr. Porges describes the vagus as having two branches, the dorsal or posterior vagus and the ventral vagal nerve complex. The ventral vagal complex, also referred to by Porges as the "social vagus," is primarily associated with the nucleus ambiguous in the brainstem and appears to be associated with social communication and self-soothing. We will be discussing this more in the next section. The dorsal vagus is thought to be older, from an evolutionary standpoint, and can produce a profound "freezing" parasympathetic influence on the nervous system, part of the fight-flight-freeze response (see figure 10.3 on page 184). The evolutionary role of the fight-flight-freeze response was to help an animal being preyed upon to survive by either fighting, fleeing, or becoming immobilized and feigning death when intense fear is present, tricking the predator and perhaps living longer. Another aspect of the dorsal vagus allows for "immobility without fear" seen in prosocial behaviors that are thought to be mediated by oxytocin, which in mammals allows for such activities such as childbirth, orgasm, and nursing and likely also contributes

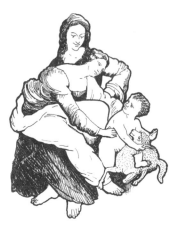 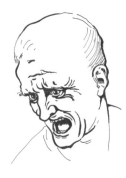 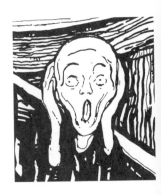

Figure 10.3. Faces showing the social vagus and fight-flight-freeze response. From left to right we see a joyful connection and play promoted by an active social vagus nerve, anger as one can experience in a fight or flee response, and then terror to point of being scared to death or fainting, which is the freeze response. Self-regulatory techniques like Kriya yoga move our nervous system more toward the social engagement side of the spectrum. (Images based on work by Leonardo Da Vinci and Edvard Munch.)

to the great stillness in deep states of meditation as well as attachment to another living being.

## Sexual Trauma and the Polyvagal Theory

The idea that sexual orgasm is something that occurs in a state of immobilization without fear is the likely reason why sexual trauma can be so challenging to treat. This is a trauma occurring at a very deep and relatively primitive level within our autonomic nervous system. When trauma occurs at this level it is beyond words. There also appears to be a sense of betrayal of the nervous system as sexual arousal, which previously had occurred only when one was feeling safe in a state of immobilization without fear now occurs entwined with fear and terror.

This type of experience can be destabilizing from the deepest level of our lived experience, as our nervous system, in a way, betrays us. The complication occurs when there is a mismatch between the deep primitive function of the autonomic nervous system—terror (immobilization with fear)—and the function of deep connection and safety (immobilization without fear). Violence perpetrated toward someone by a loved one or one whom someone is dependent on causes the same problem. As much of traumatic memory is nonverbal, somatic therapies and auricular acupuncture combined with psychotherapy can often help one reexperience some of the trauma in a state where the parasympathetic system has been encouraged to come online in a stronger fashion, providing the ground for both the verbal and nonverbal memories to begin a beneficial integration without retraumatization. It is also possible that deeper healing can occur with deep states of meditation after the somatic therapies have done all they can.

Reentering a state of immobilization without fear can still be very traumatic and even dissociative if some healing has not already occurred. This is one of the reasons any self-regulatory technique must be done carefully in a safe place and with the support of some inner resource to rely on. Often the resource is a grounded posture integrated with breath but at a more surface level than one gets to in deep meditation.

• • • • • • • • • • • • • • • • • • • • • • • • • • • • • • • • • • • • • • • • • • • • • • •

Approximately forty days after conception, an embryo is developing a rudimentary brainstem that eventually becomes the center of our autonomic nervous system (see figure 10.4 on page 186). Because this part of our brain develops first, a deep instinct for survival is deeply rooted in the base of our nervous system and comes alongside the emotional mechanisms for survival such as fear and anxiety, which are intrinsically linked to and influence our higher cognitive functions. As you can see in figure 10.4 on page 186, our higher brain structures and functions are built on the back of the more rudimentary, involuntary part of our nervous system, which is essential for survival and life-sustaining functions. When these lower centers are influenced by trauma and the chronic stress and strain of the contemporary world, they can highjack the higher cortical functions.

This is why problems with anxiety, panic, and trauma can be so overwhelming. The root of the aberrant neuronal firing begins deep in the brainstem, which in turn markedly diminishes the ability of our thinking brain, our cortex, to exert an rational influence. This is how the fight-flight-freeze response takes over as a life-saving measure during times of threat. However, when this response is triggered by something that is not a threat, it becomes a liability and needs attention to return to a more appropriate level of activation.

When our rudimentary survival and higher cortex functions are at odds with each other—for example, during a panic or anxiety attack—higher brain functions give way to the more pressing need of "make it out alive." This can become habitual and triggered by benign everyday occurrences that then interfere with our functioning. However, the

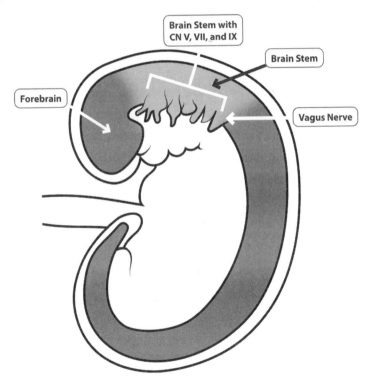

Figure 10.4. Root of the autonomic nervous system at approximately forty days gestational age

basic structure and beautiful elegance of our nervous system underpins our body's network of cells, pulsing and communicating with the rest of the system and capably moving past habitual behaviors that have developed from anxiety or trauma.

We are a resilient species capable of reinventing ourselves, which includes rewiring our brains so that past experiences have less of a hold on us and we have more choice on how to move forward on our path.

. . . . . . . . . . . . . . . . . . . . . . . . . . . . . . . . . . . . . . . . . . .

## Returning to Balance: The Importance of Sleep

To begin balancing the nervous system in general and the autonomic nervous system in particular, we need to address the importance of rest. Sleep has a profound effect on our ability to thrive and sustain health via the regulation of hormones like cortisol and melatonin. The cycle of the rising and setting of the sun guides our internal circadian rhythms and through simple, routine connections with nature, we become less susceptible to illness and more likely to thrive. Our bodies are intrinsically linked to natural cycles; for example, the morning light sends a signal to our brain that in turn sets up the circadian rhythms of the body-mind. This in turn sets up the time when melatonin will rise in the evening and make us feel sleepy. This is our body's way to tell us that it is time to sleep. Unfortunately, modern humans more often than not ignore this signal and experience a "second wind." The problem with this is that we lose melatonin's help in falling asleep and insomnia often results.

Part of our circadian rhythm also programs cortisol to rise in early morning before we awake. This time is set by our waking time and morning exposure to light the previous day. It is the cortisol that gently prepares our central nervous system to be awake. Sleeping through this natural rise in cortisol leads to feelings of sluggishness once one finally gets out of bed. When one "sleeps in," it can often feel difficult to wake up totally and feel fully engaged in that day.

Cortisol helps us function in the most basic way. An imbalance of cortisol activity is detrimental to the body and is present during chronic stress, which occurs when cortisol is chronically elevated, or its natural pattern of ebb and flow throughout the day is disrupted. Working with the natural cycles to create a routine that the body can count on allows the mind as well as the central nervous system to engage and rest more fully. It is a simple practice that helps one maintain a connection to nature.

. . . . . . . . . . . . . . . . . . . . . . . . . . . . . . . . . . . . . . . . . . . . . . . . . . . .

## KRIYA YOGA AND THE POLYVAGAL THEORY

The most interesting development in the polyvagal theory is the description of the ventral branch of the vagus nerve, or social vagus. This particular branch is myelinated, or insulated in layers of fat, to allow for more rapid communication between neurons, which can therefore carry messages more quickly than the older unmyelinated dorsal branch.

In the polyvagal theory, Dr. Porges postulates that this branch of the vagus nerve has evolved in primates to the point that is intricately related to social communication and is deeply entwined with humans' ability to feel safe, engage in socialization, and self soothe. Dr. Porges describes a system where the ventral complex of the vagal nerve is involved in monitoring and interacting with the social environment. Facial movement, head and facial gestures, vocalization, and extraneous-sound filtering all contribute to our sense of safety and our ability to socially engage with others and are influenced by a group of cranial nerves described below.

The reason we are focusing on the autonomic nervous system and in particular the parasympathetic nervous system and the vagus nerve is to gain a deeper understanding of how the contemplative arts and the practice of Kriya yoga, specifically, can help strengthen, reinforce, and increase our ability to modulate the parasympathetic nervous system and the vagus nerve and increase our resiliency and resistance to stress as well as improve our social engagement.

Self-regulatory techniques like Kriya yoga intuitively recruit aspects of the social vagus to move our nervous system more toward the social engagement side of the spectrum and help harness the power of Self-Realization. These techniques are effective because they focus on the breath, which is intimately related to the vagus nerve and has the most direct effect on our ability to experience deep physiological relaxation. The breath is our only direct route to modulate the autonomic nervous system. Our breath is unique in that we do not have to think about breathing but at the same time we can consciously change our breathing patterns and even hold our breath to the point of passing out. Because we can change the patterns of our breath so easily, it is our way to have a direct and immediate impact on the tone of our autonomic nervous system at any given time.

All self-regulatory techniques are in essence restorative processes that help to build strength and resilience within the parasympathetic nervous system, thus increasing the balance between deep physiological relaxation and activation; in other words, improving the integration of the parasympathetic and sympathetic branches of our autonomic nervous system. Heart rate variability is one such measure of this relationship: the greater the heart rate variability, the greater the ability to move in and out of various states of stress, and the healthier we are. If the parasympathetic system and vagus nerve are weak for long periods of time, one has less resilience and tends to stay in a relative state of chronic stress.

To better appreciate how Kriya yoga can influence the social vagus, it can be helpful to understand how the interaction of the cranial nerves with the autonomic and central nervous system make up the social engagement system in Dr. Porges's theory. As shown in figure 10.5 on page 190, the physical nuclei of the vagus nerve—cranial nerve, or CN 10—and some of the other cranial nerve nuclei that are associated with the polyvagal theory are in very close proximity to one another within the brainstem. They appear distinctly separate in this simplified schematic illustration. The important point to understand here is that these nerve centers in the brainstem interact with each other in a myriad of ways via a variety of feedback loops and do not exist in isolation.

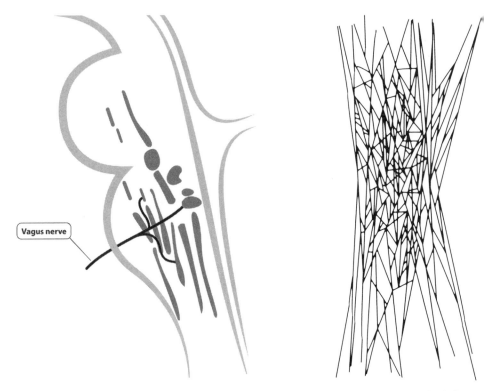

Figure 10.5. Brainstem with the cranial nerve nuclei shown in gray on the left. The right side is a stylized picture of a spider web to illustrate a somewhat exaggerated view of what the connections are like within this small area of the nervous system.

They can be thought of as more like a web of connections. This is the main home of our most basic physiological functions. This is clearly an intricate system that communicates within itself as well as with the nervous system as a whole. The polyvagal theory discusses some of this interaction and Kriya yoga makes use of this part of the brain to modulate our states of awareness.

The cranial nerves are twelve in number. We are primarily interested in those that involve Kriya: the vagus and those that overlap with vagus in function and physical proximity. The cranial nerves that are shared in both Kriya and the polyvagal theory are numbered, named, and described below. They are involved in aspects of social communication through either head and facial movements and expression, the use of voice to communicate, sound filtering as well as our breath and cardiovascular system.

- Trigeminal nerve (CN V)—The trigeminal nerve has three branches: the ophthalmic branch, the maxillary branch, and the mandibular branch. In general, they relate respectively to the sensory aspects of the upper eyelid eye, the middle and lower face, and the muscles of the jaw. This nerve also innervates the dura mater of the central nervous system.
- Facial nerve (CN VII)—The facial nerve is involved with the muscles of the face and controls facial expressions.
- Glossopharyngeal nerve (CN IX)—The glossopharyngeal nerve is involved with the function of the upper throat and the back of the tongue.
- Vagus nerve (CN X)—The vagus nerve is the root of the parasympathetic part of our autonomic nervous system and contributes to our voice box. It affects all our internal organs and their functions including our breath and heart rate.
- Accessory nerve (CN XI)—The accessory nerve controls the muscles of the neck that help turn the head from side to side and the area of the upper back where many people carry stress.

Looking at Dr. Porges's social engagement theory from the standpoint of the cranial nerves involved and their interaction with the vagus, it becomes clear that Kriya yoga is unique among the infinite number of self-regulatory techniques in that it involves breath and subtle postural exercises that touch on all aspects of the social engagement theory from the standpoint of cranial nerve involvement. These exercises and their effect on the cranial nerves are as follows:

- Practicing all the various breath-related practices has a direct influence on the vagus nerve (CN X), which directly affects the heart, the bronchi, the autonomic system in general, and the head and face in particular.

- Holding the head still and tilted slightly downward activates the neck muscles, engaging the accessory nerve (CN XI).
- Practicing ocean breath and the neck bandha engages the glottis, pharyngeal, and laryngeal muscles and thus the vagus and glossopharyngeal nerves (CNs X and IX).
- Slightly raising the eyebrows and smiling activates the facial nerve (CN VII).
- Keeping the tongue still and up against the palate quiets the feedback received by the cranial nerves that are involved in the mouth and tongue movement and chewing (CN V).
- Focusing on an inner sound or mantra decreases awareness on external sounds, potentially influencing the middle ear muscles and facial nerve (CN VII) as well.
- Practicing maha mudra, the bow, and the neck bandha puts some pressure on the dural covering of the brain and spinal cord, which is innervated by the trigeminal nerve (CN V), giving further feedback to the social engagements system.

Almost each and every practice within Kriya yoga influences the social engagement aspect of the polyvagal theory put forth by Stephen Porges, Ph.D. Together they provide a deeper understanding of the science of self-regulatory techniques and what they offer for the further psycho-spiritual evolution of humanity. Looking at Kriya yoga with the polyvagal theory, then, is another example of ancient knowledge and modern science coming together to improve our understanding of ourselves and the world in which we live.

# 11
# The Brilliant and Intelligent Brain

*Meditate and rewire your brain.*

In everyday conversation, the word *intelligence* typically refers to how "smart" somebody is. *The Merriam-Webster Dictionary* defines intelligence as "the ability to learn, understand or deal with new or trying situations; the ability to apply knowledge to manipulate one's environment or to think abstractly as measured by objective criteria such as tests." Christian Science defines intelligence as "the basic eternal quality of divine mind." Einstein is quoted as saying, "the true sign of intelligence is not knowledge, but imagination."

The psychologist Howard Gardner came up with the theory of multiple intelligences and ultimately identified eight to ten distinct types: musical, spatial, linguistic, logical-mathematical, bodily-kinesthetic, interpersonal, intrapersonal, and naturalistic, and potentially existential/spiritual as well. His theory proposes that predispositions of an individual nervous system are influenced by the input of data as much as the system's ability to identify and process that data.

Robert Sternberg put forth the triarchic theory of intelligence, advocating that an IQ test was not sufficient to determine one's level of intelligence; one also needed to look at analytical, creative, and practical intelligence. And Daniel Goleman put forth the theory of emotional intelligence, which deals more with social relatedness, self-awareness, and self-regulation. What we can glean from these forward thinkers is that intelligence is uniquely creative and that within it exists the uncanny ability to pull together disparate pieces of data and come up with a process from which new development can occur. This ultimately means we are wired to infinitely evolve and develop as a species.

Intelligence is perhaps most simply defined as "pattern recognition." We have discussed the idea that intelligence is a core feature of Nature, the human body, and the Spirit. It is posited to be found in the mind, the imagination, and perhaps every cell in the body. The central nervous system is intelligent and thereby so is the brain in its ability to rewire itself and adapt based on learning patterns. In neuroscience, this is referred to as neuroplasticity. In the past twenty-five years we've gained an understanding that certain neurons in our brain, previously thought to be nonrenewable, do in fact have the ability to regenerate themselves in certain situations. We have now seen pictures of neurons that physically change in response to environmental stimuli (see figure 11.1). There's also increased understanding of the disastrous and negative effects that trauma and deprivation have on a young nervous system and what an improved environment that is nonviolent, predictable, and sustainable can do to help a system that is struggling.

Our brain is the organ responsible for mediating millions of bits of information coming into the system, and while it is certainly an intriguing organ, it is not really a single organ as we typically think of it. It would be much more accurate to think of the brain as a number of different organs that happened to grow up and evolve together inside a skull and had to learn to work together. The brain consists of three basic parts: the cortex, which is the thinking part; the limbic system, or emotional center; and the brainstem, often called the reptilian brain, which consists of the autonomic nervous system. For this

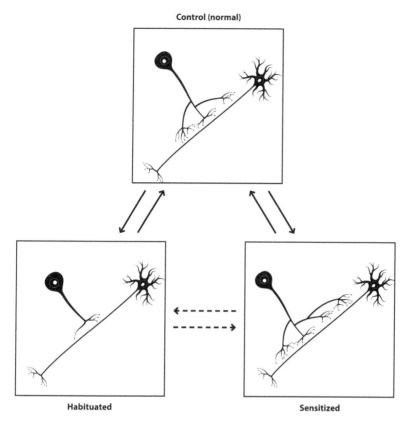

Figure 11.1. This figure illustrates how an individual neuron can grow more or resorb preexisting connections to other neurons depending upon the stimulus in the environment.

reason, we refer to it as a "triune" brain (see figure 11.2 on page 196).*

The actual breakdown is far more complex than this, but these three systems allow connections throughout the body and each plays a particular role. As discussed in the previous chapter, these systems don't always work in harmony as one can override the other depending on events in the environment. One example is the fight-flight-freeze

---

*The idea of the triune brain correlates with evolution as reptiles function primarily at the brainstem level with a primitive cortex and mammals have a functioning limbic system and are clearly able to resonant on an emotion level. Primates and potentially some cetaceans have a more developed cortex allowing for more complex thought. Once again there is overlap as this is a broad but helpful way to look at the structure of the nervous system.

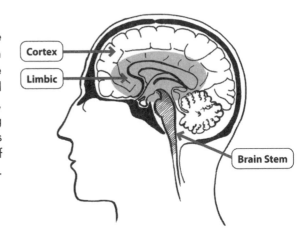

Figure 11.2. *Triune brain,* a term first used in the 1960s by Paul D. MacLean, M.D., is a way of looking at our brain as being composed of three different parts.

response described in the previous chapter. When this response is triggered the cognitive or thinking part of the brain function is decreased as the body mobilizes a survival response. Our cortex goes offline so to speak, as there is no time to think, only react. The ability to flee, fight back, faint, or play dead has proven to be a crucial survival mechanism for many species. Unfortunately, in contemporary society the many threats, perceived or imagined tend to give rise to more chronic survival responses that increase the level of stress hormones in the body, as well as arousal, anxiety, and fear. In fight or flight responses we may identify with bits of data that pose a threat and take action toward what we deem to be safety, but trauma is based partly on perception and memories that do not always serve us.

When we experience a traumatic event like a car accident or assault, it generally happens so quickly that our ability to understand it with language is turned off as we are attempting to survive. These experiences remain with us in an implicit body memory and the ability to fully recall the situation with words is limited. For this reason, talk therapies often require additional components to help people transcend traumas. Techniques that integrate body memory with explicit/verbal and autobiographical memory can be remarkably healing in some situations. This occurs by recruiting the autonomic nervous system and brain to speak "online" at the same time that the explicit or narrative memory is engaging with the unconscious body memories. When this happens, if anxiety and terror are not overwhelming for the individual, reintegration can begin to occur, the information can be processed in a new way and remembered with much less emotional charge.

Trauma and anxiety tend to lock the nervous system in a state of dysregulation where a seemingly benign stimulus either becomes increasingly disturbing or goes completely unnoticed due to hyper- or hypoarousal states that occur after trauma. This is also a problem with chronic stress. A deep-seated memory, if developed at the time of stress when the brain is awash with stress hormones, helps us remember what things to avoid next time, but if triggered continually can block the formation of new memories and cause health concerns. This can also inhibit the person's ability to talk about the trauma, which is an inherent problem in the treatment of it. Trauma and anxiety also interrupt the process with which we decipher input. For example, if there is a sound coming from another room or down the road it may not register as anything worth noting. If it were a loud sound it is more likely that the mind would consider it and decide if it is worrisome or not, depending on the environment. If the individual hearing this sound perceives the sound as one that is threatening because they have become sensitized to it, the noise itself will increase stress hormones and send the individual's central nervous system into a state of hyperarousal. These perpetually negative emotions trigger a wash of hormones that teach the cells of the brain to be on alert and eventually the functionality of the entire system is negatively affected.

Often this pattern develops after chronic stress or an acute life-threatening situation, which can also lead to the development of PTSD. These conditions blur the lines between what is real and what is not as an individual is stretched beyond their natural capacity to find balance. These are extreme examples of stress and anxiety, but we experience lesser ones every day that negatively affect our ability to correctly assess a situation, react appropriately, and decompress from stress without being compounded by past reactions and experiences. The skills that allow one to help manage chronic stressors are no longer part of daily experience in most parts of the world. In the West, individuals are under continual and mounting stress from employment, bills, or the pursuit of the latest hedonistic pleasure. The ability to allow our nervous systems to regulate is hindered by distractions, games, movies, screen time, and perpetual fear of one threat or other.

In nearly every country on Earth there are natural disasters, war, crime, famine, or unrest that constantly threaten the well-being of its citizens. In these conditions it is very difficult to experience joy or contentment, calm or restfulness, and understanding the deep healing potential of breath becomes more important than ever. Without the ability to find a deep mode of relaxation that allows our nervous systems to regenerate and move forward with creative resources, we become more fragile and fractured individuals and contribute those same characteristics to the global society.

These multidimensional effects of chronic stress on the body and society are still active areas of research. What we do know is that the brain is chemically altered by stress hormones and over time those hormones change the physiology of the brain by changing the interneuronal connections. Long-term stress decreases the ability to acquire new information, impeding an individual's ability to learn or memorize. Memory is a form of learning and has been essential to our species' survival. It is how we have evolved to this point. The neurons within the brain communicate and through their communication develop a variety of efficiencies based on intelligent pattern recognition. For example, when viewing the brain activity of someone learning a new skill, we can see that the individual is harnessing a tremendous amount of central nervous system real estate to analyze a problem. An expert in the subject, however, requires much less memory (space in the cortex) or resources to complete the task (see figure 11.3). This pattern of learning happens in meditation as well. A beginner can take days, months, or years to reach the same place an experienced meditator can enter in seconds. This is the nature of our intelligence and how practice leads to expertise.

Intelligence is not quarantined in the brain but is in fact present within every cell of the body. The body remembers its experiences too. A wonderful development in psychotherapy in recent decades includes the rise of somatic psychotherapies such as bioenergetics, formative psychology, the Hakomi Method, and eye movement desensitization and reprocessing, or EMDR, that came out of the work of Wilhelm Reich, Alexander Lowen, Stanley Keleman, Ron Kurtz, and Francine Shapiro, respectively.

In recent years Joseph M. Helms, M.D. and Richard C. Niemtzow, M.D., Ph.D. of the U.S. Air Force developed auricular acupuncture techniques that directly recruit the autonomic nervous system. They found that by placing acupuncture needles in specific locations on the ear and then discussing the traumas lead to remarkable improvement in PTSD symptoms and acute pain.

Neuroplasticity is arguably the most important evolutionary aspect of any nervous system. The term refers to the ability of our nerves to be "plastic," or pliable, and allows for a constant state of change, which is what enables us to learn. Learning, or as it is technically known, "long-term potentiation," involves physical changes within our brain. New physical connections are made in order to meet the demand of storing a new pattern of information that needs to be remembered. Trivial experiences don't necessarily get remembered long-term but traumatic

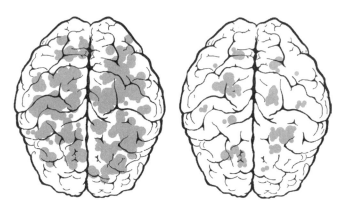

Figure 11.3. This figure represents a beginner on the left and an experienced individual on the right. The gray areas represent the activation of the neurons. While the two brains are both engaged in the same task, the experienced brain is utilizing less energy and resources to complete it.

memories do, as does anything we repeat a few times in short order and also begin using right away.

Learning is influenced by internal and external stimuli, which include what is happening at the moment, what happened last year, and what happened in childhood. An ongoing area of research called epigenetics even suggests that some of this information can be transmitted from parents' experiences and passed to offspring. For instance, when a child is born into a family where one or both parents are struggling with depression and anxiety, the stress and subsequent trauma is transferred to the younger generation and sometimes many generations after that until the pattern is finally broken.

But while it is well accepted that learned behavior is passed down through generations, it now seems that it may even imprint our genes to change how they function and respond to stressors in the environment. It is well accepted by science that the eating patterns of your grandparents have been shown to have an effect on how genes related to physical illness are expressed in you, two generations later, which is an example of epigenetics. The implications of this research suggest that if a method for prevention of psychological trauma and chronic stress can be learned by one generation, it can be passed down through future generations. So not only can these practices help somebody who is on the verge of exhaustion and burnout today, they can also lead to improved resilience, better functioning, and less reactivity to bouts of stress for generations to come.

In just one generation this could have a huge impact on a population in general and help us move toward a more prosocial, supportive society and away from one that is highly isolated, anxious, fearful, and angry. If the world's educational system included the teaching of self-regulatory techniques it would go a long way toward breaking up some of the intergenerational transfers of trauma. This could easily occur as we see various types of self-regulatory techniques becoming more embedded in society. Mental health professionals are becoming more aware of these methods, and if this continues, we will begin to see positive changes in the future.

# PART IV

# THE SPIRITUAL EFFECTS OF KRIYA YOGA

# 12

# Survival of the
# Most Mindful

*Joy is when Spirit touches the body and mind
with a glimpse of the Infinite.*

Health in the broadest sense is the ability to self-regulate, so self-regulation is the foundation of wellness. Getting the most basic aspects of life in balance provides a structure from which to grow and branch out. It is important to move forward with the practice of self-regulatory techniques and begin to think of life as an opportunity to take action toward wellness. Health isn't just simply the absence of disease; rather, it is a spectrum that continually evolves. With improved physical functioning comes a greater sense of joy and connection with others and with nature, both of which can be very healing.

Despite current detrimental behaviors running rampant in the United States and across the globe, humans are hardwired for joy. We cannot otherwise explain the bliss of spiritual experiences described by spiritual leaders for millennia. One can think of joy as the moment when Spirit touches the body and mind with a glimpse of the Infinite. The first step to moving along this pathway to joy is decreasing the impacts of toxic stress on the body through spinal awareness; full, regular, reposed, rhythmic respiration; cognitive flexibility; altruistic compassion; and tuning in to the cycles of nature that surrounds us.

Until recently, the Western viewpoint of psychology focused more on the mind as a "house of obstacles." The emphasis tended to be more on pathology, i.e., looking for repression and resistance and finding problems that needed to be "fixed." The unconscious was often seen as dark source of angst, an unknown and at times an infinite challenge to unearth and bring into the light of day. Mindful awareness and the work of Kriya, however, assist the mind in expanding beyond preconceived limitations to allow for a greater sense of wellness overall.

One Western psychologist who looked at well-being from an Eastern perspective was Abraham Maslow. In 1943, he began work on a theory he described as the "hierarchy of needs." He continued to revise this theory until his death in 1970. His initial work looked at five tiers of human needs: physiological (food, water, warmth, rest), safety (security), belongingness and love (intimate relationships/ sex and friends), esteem (feelings of accomplishment), and self-actualization (achieving one's full potential). He did not, however, include Self-Realization, as his work stopped with the idea of self-actualization, which refers more to reaching one's full potential from a physiological and psychological standpoint rather than a spiritual one. The theory did, however, significantly expand ideas of development within psychology.

Ganesh Baba's theory was developed during the same years and is similar in that for the majority of people neither psychological well-being or spiritual development could occur until one's basic physiological needs were met. Ganesh Baba looked at this issue from the standpoint of evolution basing his views on Darwin's model of the survival of the fittest. Those who are able to survive physically are then able to move forward with psychological and spiritual evolution. Therefore, the groups that were best adapted to the environment survived and went on to procreate.

The main point here is that until one's physical needs get met, it is very difficult to move beyond survival mode. We become distracted by the need for sustenance, shelter, security, and sex, and especially during times of stress, our ability to nurture social connectedness, build esteem, or develop and sustain greater awareness is limited. Only when we feel secure from a survival of the fittest standpoint can we make significant gains with self-regulation, self-integration, self-organization, and finally, Self-Realization.

What Ganesh Baba referred to as S1–S4 was largely based on Darwinian evolution as shown in the list below. Ganesh Baba identified the basic survival needs as shelter, sex, sustenance, and security. These needs also correspond to the yoga idea of the chakras (see figure 8.8 on page 146) and what they represent while at the same time corresponding to the idea of fertilization of an egg in reproduction. As discussed in previous chapters, the first chakra (S1), beginning at the base of the spine, or the coccyx, is the root chakra and is associated with our connection the earth and shelter. The second, or sacral chakra (S2), is associated with reproduction. The third chakra (S3) is in the lumbar area, our abdomen, and is associated with fire and absorption of nutrients. Finally, the thoracic, or heart, chakra (S4) is associated with compassion, connection, and security. These are presented in a hierarchical order with the root chakra needing to be established first before sex, food, and security in that order as shown in the list below.

GANESH BABA'S S1-S4 THEORY AND THE CHAKRAS

S1—Shelter: coccyx root/earth chakra
S2—Sex: sacral chakra
S3—Sustenance: lumbar chakra
S4—Security: thoracic heart chakra

There is also an interesting correspondence here with sexual reproduction and child development. If we look at conception and begin with the sperm entering the egg, a place of shelter (S1) where it can begin to live and that corresponds to the root chakra. The sperm's next function is to fertilize the egg and share genetic material (S2), which corresponds to the sacral/genital chakra. The fertilized egg begins growth by cell division and moves into the uterus where it initially absorbs some nutrition from the immediate environment (S3), which represents the lumbar chakra. It then proceeds with implantation into the safe, nutrient rich, and secure (S4) environment of the uterus. This stage represents the heart chakra. The environment around the egg provides nine months of security while the fetus continues to grow. Here one can imagine that a sense of belonging and a deep sense of connection develop and the connection to the heart chakra can easily be drawn.

When birth occurs, the fetus moves out and into its next phase of life where it begins to communicate with the outside world, which correlates to the cervical/throat chakra associated with speech and language. Initially any sounds made here are associated with survival and correlate more to the first three chakras. Once the child begins to bond with the parents we see once again the heart chakra engaged, and once the child begins to talk, we then have the cervical/throat chakra being activated. As one can see the philosophical ideas behind the chakras have real resonance with human development and evolution. It is then up to the individual to move forward to higher levels of development.

To further build upon this idea, Ganesh Baba and I worked together and developed the ideas of S5–S8 (see the list below). This continues the corollary with what Ganesh Baba liked to call *psychozoic* evolution to refer to the epoch in evolutionary time since modern humans arrived and established themselves as "fit" enough to survive in the world.

### GANESH BABA'S PSYCHOZOIC EVOLUTION

S5—Self-evaluation: psychological reflection; intra/interpersonal awareness, refinement, and development; manual on/off control of parts

S6—Self-regulation: mind-body integration (V1–V2); intrapersonal awareness, refinement, and development; integration of parts, like a thermostat

S7—Self-integration: psychological integration (V3–V4); transpersonal awareness, refinement, and development; integration of systems

S8—Self-organization: meditation, emergent transcendence, emergent properties from systems reorganization

S∞—Self-realization: transcendence

We will now go through each of the S5–S8 stages one at a time beginning with self-evaluation (S5). This stage of development is not unique to Kriya, and it is also related to Patanjali's yoga sutras. It includes the yamas and niyamas, which means we are beginning to know better but are still striving to achieve. This stage represents a point in development where one is beginning to feel safe and connected with others in a more socially cohesive fashion and allows for self-evaluation and a sense of belonging. However, since this state can easily be disrupted with a stressor, it acts more like an on-off switch initially.

With time this change naturally leads to down regulation of the fight-or-flight response, and deeper physiological relaxation can then occur, which in turns brings awareness to the breath and posture. This physiological change in reactivity is the beginning of Kriya yoga. As posture and breath (V1 and V2) are developed and practiced, there is a noticeable a shift in function.

Self-regulation (S6) includes the point when the posture and breath aspects of Kriya yoga have been experienced and have been practiced regularly for a period of time. This is the beginning of gaining mastery over one's own body and mind in an integrated fashion. At this point one has managed to set up a thermostat within with regard to self-regulation. It involves working with the limbic system, our emotional center, and creating a new set point. This is the path to limbic integration where reactivity becomes less of a presence. The thermostat works in most situations, and we begin to automatically follow a new more integrated path in our thoughts and interactions with others. This is the point where we begin to have a deeper understanding of just how interrelated the mind, emotions, and breath are.

Self-integration (S7) refers to the next two phases of Kriya yoga previously referred to as visualization (V3) and vibrationalization (V4). These two phases include a retraction of the outward visual and auditory senses toward an inner focus and with time the beginning stages of meditation. This is a phase where one experiences an integration of various systems from new learned behaviors and practices. Our higher levels of cognition are becoming more involved at this level and are more readily available. Neuroplastic changes in one system meet and connect with neuroplastic changes in another system, and the communication between the two systems begins to function at new levels, encouraging emergent properties to take hold through the association areas of the cortex. At this point in time, a new persona begins to emerge within the individual. While their personality does not change, it integrates and becomes more radiant and compassionate and holds much less baggage, as it now recognizes the transpersonal connection.

The final phase of this system before Self-Realization is self-organization (S8), which represents the new emergent properties of meditation. A functional change is established from the previous level of system integration and comes with new levels of awareness and a sense of connectedness with the whole. Inter-, intra-, and transpersonal levels are now integrated and internalized as a recognized whole and are no longer experienced as separate parts. Compassion is now fully integrated into daily function and is rarely if ever disrupted.

Once one is able to obtain and maintain self-regulation, self-integration, and self-organization, Self-Realization beckons. This final step S∞, is the attainment of Knowledge and the unified experience of Consciousness. At this phase one's whole body, mind, and spirit have experienced a new reality due to emergent change within the systems, and Self-Realization occurs. This leaves long lasting neuroplastic changes in one's central nervous system.

This system of S1–S8 is an attempt to delineate the biological, psychological, and spiritual evolution of an individual with a meditative practice as they move beyond basic survival toward Self-Realization. This is a theoretical construct like the Cycle of Synthesis. Both are attempts to give clarity and structure to the idea of psychospiritual integration so that additional work can occur in this area as we move forward in our collective evolution. These theories are an effort to reinforce the idea that once human beings' physiological needs are met, a more meaningful evolution is possible and necessary. At this point psychological and spiritual development is essential for survival and the experience of joy.

The path from S1–S4 to S5–S8 can be easily disrupted at least in the beginning stages. This can be seen almost anywhere in the world when any of the S1–S4 survival needs are not met. Having some embodiment of higher levels of psychospiritual integration does allow a good degree of resiliency when dealing with the trauma and stressors that are currently occurring on a global scale. Be present, be mindful, and practice, practice, practice, and share what you learn when the opportunity presents itself.

## THE FOURFOLD PATH OF STRIVING

The psychospiritual integration that occurs with the contemplative arts is a specific integration process that can be demonstrated through what Ganesh Baba taught as the Fourfold Path of Striving. These are stages that begin in earnest when one begins to meditate and thus correspond to the seventh aspect, dhyana/meditation, of Patanjali's yoga sutras.

There are four distinct stages of attainment as one moves forward and strives for health and spiritualization. The first stage is the consideration of impermanence where one comes to understand and accept the movement of life, death, cycles, and change. The second stage is the embodiment of nonattachment. The third stage is the acquisition of the six spiritual wealths. The fourth stage is the aspiration to salvation.

### Stage 1: Consideration of Impermanence

As one gains insight into what is real and unreal, what is permanent and perishable, one begins to understand that the physical world is a world of permanent impermanence. The cycle of birth and death is ongoing for the cosmos as well as for the smallest insect. It is the absolute that is permanent and all sustaining and permeates everything. This insight comes from contemplation. This is the first true insight that allows one to see our infinite dimension that is beyond time. It should not be taken on "blind faith" but instead experienced through one's own practice. Unfortunately, with time blind faith can move one toward insecurity, anger, and agnosticism. On the other hand, if one can taste the permanence of the absolute, faith flowers throughout one's being.

This seed needs care as without it the bombardment of the physical universe can lead to the spiritual insight being forgotten. Relapsing into old habits in times of stress or boredom can occur. In the current materialistic civilization this process can be hard and one needs to take care to nurture their insight and heart's desires. When one begins to experience changes in their outlook they also experience shifts in personality and a blossoming of spiritual wisdom. However, one does not lose focus on education, livelihood, or secular duties, and Kriya yoga teaches the householder to maintain their role in society.

### Stage 2: Embodiment of Nonattachment

This stage may only be possible once one has come to terms with impermanence. A sense of what is impermanent in the cosmos allows one to begin the slow, steady development of positive detachment. There is a greater sense of equanimity. Surrender to a higher order brings a new kind of security and there is less need for distraction, less disturbance in one's life. There is an increased awareness and development of an internal versus an external sense of authority. Surrender and positive detachment are difficult concepts for some to comprehend. Neither concept promotes the practitioner giving up their own sense of self in order to know true spiritual power. They merely ask that trust be practiced with an open curiosity for change. A balanced approach to action and thought will help one release an attachment to a specific outcome. In doing so, one finds a distinct internal level of freedom unknown to mainstream society.

### Stage 3: Acquisition of Six Spiritual Wealths

As outlined by Ganesh Baba these six qualities are experiences along the path to Self-Realization. These wealths are realized through intuitive introspection and meditative practice and represent a path toward spiritual evolution. With a daily Kriya practice one can expect to have these experiences. It is with the regulation of breath and these exercises that infinite resources are provided to the practitioner.

### First Spiritual Wealth: Forbearance and Equanimity (Shama)

The capacity to maintain one's focus on the spiritual path despite distracted impulses of anger, lust, greed, arrogance, hate, shyness, fear, or self-protection. The ability to do this on a consistent basis is referred to as forbearance. With the practice of Kriya one moves toward Self-Realization in the slow but consistent speed where the ability to maintain equanimity naturally takes hold and becomes one's foundation.

### Second Spiritual Wealth: Self-Regulation and Self-Restraint (Dama)

This area refers to one's ability to help manage the externally focused senses including the mind, intellect, and ego. If the practitioner is feeling overpowered they can shift within and activate what's been learned in Kriya to completely subjugate their rebellious instincts. When the student is able to succeed in these techniques, they have obtained this level of spiritual wealth.

## Third Spiritual Wealth: Firmness against Obstacles (Titikshya)

This stage has to do with ignoring obstacles along the path toward spiritualization. The aspirant now becomes unshakable, like a mountain. Impulses do not distract from the path of striving. One is able to ignore impediments without internal conflicts.

## Fourth Spiritual Wealth: Sense of Unity (Uparati)

Fellowship toward the equality of all where one experiences a deep affinity for all life and sees others as no different from oneself with compassion for all living beings. Behavior becomes benign and any malcontent is swept away by one's own awakened heart. No hatred or animosities are harbored while none are excluded. One might consider this a place of balance worth striving for.

## Fifth Spiritual Wealth: Sincere and Deep Regard for the Well-Being of All (Shraddha)

Confidence in universality. Respect for life becomes deeper and more pervasive. As one takes steps of appreciation and respect for the path that they're on, deep regard emerges. The experience of consciousness deepens through the regular practice of Kriya. Without this appreciation for the gifts that one has received, the breath of Kriya can remain fairly superficial.

## Sixth Spiritual Wealth: Solution/Knowledge Doubtlessness (Samadhana)

The clarity of understanding. Here the practitioner experiences the totality of Knowledge as diverse. As Ganesh Baba said, there is a "floodlight of omniscience, no darkness or doubt remains." One now begins to experience altruistic love and infinite compassion for all beings.

One becomes "doubt free." This is the state preceding the final state of enlightenment, liberation, and true salvation known as samadhi.

## Stage 4: Aspiration to Salvation

This final stage is a deep desire for liberation. Once in this state, Indian scripture describes, rebirths and incarnations will no longer need to occur. This marks the end of a human experience on the earthly plane and is said to be a desire of the guru or master. Absolute existence in pure consciousness is experienced.

With the regular practice of Kriya all of the benefits of improved intra- and interpersonal traits as described in the yamas/niyamas as well as the six spiritual wealths can be obtained. In each of these moments that move us beyond survival mode and toward integration, we can foster a stronger sense of self and a deeper resonance of health and wellness. When we enhance our ability to engage in socioemotional communication in a calm and relaxed manner, we become more available to compassion and active listening and expand our tolerances. When we can see ourselves in the "other" and see the other in ourselves we become more aware of the plight of the planet, its animals, and our environment and make positive changes to afford sustainability for all involved.

Interpersonal and intrapersonal intelligence improves the ability to reflect, but it also improves our ability to manage survival instincts that focus on security, sustenance, shelter, and sex and move more gracefully toward spiritualization. The spirituality of yoga is all encompassing and recognizes that all spirituality is the same; it does not see yogis as any more advanced, superior, or enlightened than Buddhist monks, Sufi practitioners, Christian mystics, practitioners of Kabbalah, or any other path that leads to Self-Realization. When practiced regularly Kriya will stimulate innate intelligence to evolve toward an experience of the unified whole and offer foundational wellness. Health then, is the ability to become more integrated in body and mind, more agile, and more capable of experiencing joy until the Absolute is realized with Spirit.

# 13

# Samadhi

---

*The Guru/Teacher is within.*

---

Samadhi, satori, Nirvana. . . . These are all terms from different traditions used to describe increasing awareness and the embodiment of the Absolute. Samadhi begins with one-pointed concentration, transitions through meditation, and then moves onward through various states of increasing awareness of the nature of the Absolute. Ultimately it culminates in an experience of the Absolute where one's individual sense of self merges with the Absolute Self, such that all boundaries vanish in the interconnectedness of everything that ever was and ever will be. It is at that moment that there is a brilliance beyond brilliance radiating within and without and in-between for infinity, as it knows nothing less than oneness.

It is the experience of the infinity of everything as being connected synchronistically at every moment, for all time. Every point, if there was such a thing, is communicating with every other point in an infinite fashion while at the same time there is absolute stillness and a deep sense of connection. The ultimate nonduality from which we have come, from where we are now, and to where we are going is beyond human need, emotional limitations, or mental restlessness. It is returning to a home you never knew you had. It is the deepest embodiment we are capable of while in this body. It is a way to communicate with our ultimate mother and father, namely Nature and Spirit. Through that energy a direct connection is made to the Absolute, the Godhead, the point of U3, where there is unification of All that there is and All that there ever was and All that there ever will be.

It is understood by master practitioners that human consciousness is fragmented; we are not able to sustain one-pointed focus without significant practice and intention. This is the struggle of the mind, but these transcendent states of one-pointed focus are a gift worth working for. It is through our unification of the mind with greater awareness that we begin to understand how peace is found within the journey of life. That said, samadhi is not necessarily a destination to seek, for it is the journey that has the greatest value. When we strive to imbibe each moment as a blessing, samadhi is the blessing that will find us. Samadhi is a liberation of Consciousness, and it is the experience of U3.

There are various shades or states of samadhi with one level blending with and preparing for the next. As one begins to develop the ability for one pointedness and their concentration and awareness begin to shift, a deeper sense of contemplation begins, often coinciding with a sense of compassion for self and others. As one's practice moves forward one's ability to meditate continues to progress, and these states become available without any particular one-pointed focus. At this point one's attachment to the worldly focus of survival and physical pleasures noticeably changes toward an absorption with the Absolute and a Knowledge that begins to grow regarding the more subtle aspects of human awareness. Ultimately the perceptual change shifts even further and the sense of being an individual melts to the point of barely being perceptible. At this point the totality and the lack of boundary from within and without predominates.

The various stages of Patanjali's yoga sutras and Kriya yoga (see figure 4.2 on page 52) provide a useful way to look at the various levels of samadhi experiences. The first such glimpse of samadhi (*savikalpa*) begins with Kriya level V4, or dharana, the sixth limb of Patanjali's system. As we move into this stage we are focusing on the inner sound, and contemplation begins to develop.

One-pointedness concentration is required for V4 to be able to do its work of integration. In this stage one experiences contemplation, a sense of the subtle body, and transcendence. It is often associated with a sense of liberation, reflection, and joy. This beginning stage of one-pointedness concentration allows one to engage in and appreciate the physiological changes of altruistic love that are deep and all pervading. Reflection, thoughts, and analysis can still be present to some degree but become less evident as one reenters these levels of consciousness over time. The more time one spends in these levels of awareness, the more hardwired one's central nervous system becomes to moving along the path to get there. With time, when a practitioner sits down to practice, they will find themselves in the meditation stage within moments of closing their eyes.

Once one's posture, breath, visualization, and sound have all been mastered as foci of concentration and have been synchronized and are working together, one moves toward Patanjali's seventh stage, referred to as "meditation," or dhyana, and known as *asamprajnata* samadhi (also called *nirvikalpa* samadhi), or conditional samadhi.

From this point forward the meditation takes on its own unique and creative course as one rides it through various stages of mind, intelligence, and consciousness to the Absolute. This begins as the stage of meditation without an object. It is still conditional, meaning it has yet to pervade and take on a life of its own, but that experience is on the horizon. In this realm there is an increase in Knowledge and an increase in awareness of the energetic body. One is moving toward pure Consciousness and experiences fleeting insights with regard to what that is. Although this experience is still conditional, requiring some setup for the process, the physiological states that are experienced leave lasting indelible impressions in one's psyche such that the experience of the world is no longer the same.

The eighth limb of Patanjali's system, *sahaja* samadhi, is unconditional. It is at this point in meditation where one perceives the fabric of the essence, and the Intelligence of Absolute Consciousness is revealed. The sense of being an individual melts to the point of barely being noticeable; one only perceives the totality and the lack of boundary from within and without. There is no longer an inside or an outside, an I or thou; it is all one engagement. It is the Absolute; it is the moment where inhalation and exhalation meet and are joyous in their connection as they celebrate creation and evolution in unison, and all is one, as there is no separation.

Once experience occurs in this realm it is impossible to return back to previous levels of behavior as the pervasive oneness of all of Nature and Spirit has been seen with such clarity that one has a deep visceral understanding that there is no difference between one's individual self and the cosmos or one's individual self and someone else's. This is the ultimate understanding that humans need to experience in order to move forward on the ladder of evolution away from tribal and territorial bickering to a celebration of the overwhelming beauty that this view provides as an enticement to look deeper and experience the Spirit in Nature that is all around.

Although a variety of specific states are described above, the path to samadhi is a continuum, and hard divisions rarely exist. Words are a limiting factor when describing the ineffable. The names are included as a reference to compare with other writings if you are so inclined. Be aware that it is very easy to get lost in the semantics here, but that is mind/self pursuing philosophy and religion and not our consciousness/Self exploring spirituality. It is the general ideas that are important, and the regularity of practice that is the most important of all.

Some interpretations of Buddhism allude to the idea that unconditional samadhi is not liberation and that liberation only comes through further reflection and work. It is my opinion that the jump from the seventh stage to the eighth stage of Patanjali's system is a quantum shift and includes all aspects of liberation as described in the mindfulness/ insight meditation literature. There is a lot of room for contemplation between the fifth stage and the seventh stage of Patanjali's system, where various levels of insight can be gained, but once one reaches the eighth stage, one is beyond the intermediate stages where the reflections described in insight meditation have relevance. However, they are certainly relevant while traveling along the path, taking stops, returning and retracing steps, reflecting, processing, and integrating all these aspects of increasing insight into the nature of the Absolute. In fact, it is only because we have these abilities to pause, reflect, and remember that any writings are available at all regarding these states. One can move in and out of stages five through seven throughout any meditative session. With increasing time, however, one spends less time at those levels on return visits as there is no need to retrace one's steps. The mind and the Spirit know where to go and it takes an experienced practitioner no time to return.

The eighth stage, on the other hand, is embodied Knowledge that never leaves, and if one were to live in that state perpetually, one's ability to do the laundry and wash the dishes would be somewhat limited. Thus, this stage is best suited to only be *visited* by those who are still in their years of working and raising a family and can be returned to as they move toward renunciation, as a place to dwell and provide guidance and solace for those younger individuals trotting along the path toward true Knowledge.

# 14

# Subtle Energies of Kriya

*Kriya is to be experienced. It is an embodied practice. Feel it.*

The subtle energies of Kriya yoga become apparent rather quickly. Just improving one's posture shifts one's awareness and respirations. There is immediate improvement in energy and concentration and the sense of feeling lighter and more engaged with oneself and the world around you. As one continues to practice, one becomes more aware of the subtle energies of prana within one's breath along with other subtle energies that shift the focus within the third eye. That said, the ultimate goal in Kriya yoga is to "magnetize" or "tune" the central nervous system, the brain and the spinal cord, such that it functions as an antenna for these subtle energies that are just outside the perception of our five gross senses of touch, taste, smell, sight, and hearing. As you read further on in this section, you'll be introduced to some of the anatomy of the central nervous system that is associated with these perceptual changes as well as a more detailed review of the chakras and kundalini.

As science moved forward in the early 1900s, it became clear to Ganesh Baba that it was time to merge the properties of science with the deep philosophy of Vedanta, tantra, and the techniques of yoga. This was not a huge leap forward as Ganesh Baba was first taught yoga by Swami Sivananda, who was a medical doctor. With a broad British education in the arts, science, and mathematics, Ganesh Baba was able to integrate Eastern and Western ideas into a meaningful philosophical framework to help Western and Eastern minds see the connection. Ganesh Baba's other goal was to simplify the practice as much as possible by removing cultural overtones so that no matter what one's belief system was it would not get in the way of practicing the basic physiological techniques of yogic meditation that have the potential to bring about profound and lasting changes in mind, body, and spirit integration.

This idea of integrating Western and Eastern philosophies and science with yogic meditation was presented earlier in the Cycle of Synthesis. Ganesh Baba developed these ideas in the 1950s and 1960s yet they remain relevant to our understanding of the science of creation and evolution with the contemplative sciences like meditation and the experience of Self-Realization.

Another layer of integration is that Kriya yoga utilizes various physical exercises that provide awareness and activate aspects of the central nervous system, including the spinal cord. There is a correlation here to kundalini energy as it relates to physical structures of central nervous system and the structural aspects of the spine. Engaging in various physical activities including lumbar mobilization provides some additional motion on the spinal column and, therefore, the dura mater and the cerebrospinal fluid as well. Any practitioner of cranial osteopathy can also attest to the remarkable changes that can occur to one's physiology through the subtle manipulation of these central nervous system structures.

The dura mater is one of three meninges,* It is the thickest of the meninges and is a leather-like fibrous tissue that is fascia like

---

*The three meninges are the dura mater, the arachnoid, and the pia mater. We are primarily focused on the dura here although it has a working relation with the other two. Although the dura mater is not technically considered fascia it is a thick membranous structure. All of our organs are encased in fascia with the heart and lungs having rather thick coverings. Fasica is ubiquitous throughout the body, but its role in health is only beginning to be understood. The fascia may very well be the carrier of much more information inside the body than we are aware of and dura mater may be similar. Acupuncture is one discipline that may be working via the fascia, as is cranial osteopathy.

in its structure. The meninges encase the spinal cord and the brain (see figure 14.1), protecting the central nervous system and holding it in place within its skeletal covering. Inside the cranium, the dura mater attaches to the upper part of the ethmoid bone as well as the sphenoid bone, which holds the pituitary gland and other parts of the skull. The dura mater is innervated by the branches of the fifth cranial nerve, also known as the trigeminal nerve, and nerves from the cervical region. The dura mater is watertight and keeps the neurologic tissue of the brain and spinal cord suspended in the cerebrospinal fluid, which provides nutrients, absorbs and gets rid of waste products, allows the brain to float by adding buoyancy to the organ, and provides a cushion against trauma.

Traditional Kriya yoga primarily uses maha mudra as an exercise to engage the spine and abdomen. The spinal cord is part of our brain and keeping it in good health and alignment is necessary for deep uncomplicated meditation experiences. In reflecting on the phys-

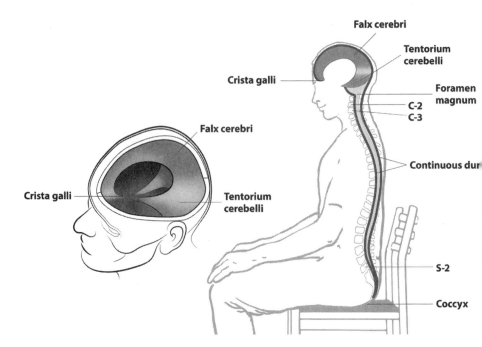

Figure 14.1. Dura mater and the central nervous system.

iology of the spinal cord it becomes clear that the various exercises influence the central nervous system via the meninges/dura mater, from the coccyx to the deep aspects of the brain, spinal cord, and cerebrospinal fluid.

Cerebrospinal fluid is made within the deep ventricles of the brain by the choroid plexus and slowly circulates throughout the brain and spinal cord, even filling the central canal, which, as you may remember, is the width of a pin and runs through the center of the spinal cord. Through various exercises and stretching activities including lumbar mobilization, motion is induced within these living membranous structures and likely influences the dura mater and the flow patterns of the cerebrospinal fluid. As this system is one continuous link it is possible to consider that shifts may occur in the central nervous system as these movements act on the meninges as a whole and inspire changes in the dynamics of cerebrospinal fluid, which can influence experience in deep meditation. As we work with conscious awareness of the physical body we may become more aware of the causal and energetic anatomy as it is refined to be a clear receptor for subtle physiological and psychological shifts.

Cranial osteopathy is a technique that was first developed by Dr. William Sutherland in the 1930s. The basis of this technique is to work with the rhythm of the cranial sacral oscillation, which is the expansion and contraction, or flexion and extension, of the central nervous system within its skeletal, meningeal, and fascial enclosure. The work is focused around what osteopathy calls the primary respiratory mechanism, but this is not the inhalation and exhalation that happens when one takes a breath. Rather, it is a flexion and extension of the body as a whole, emanating from the central nervous system. Through careful observation, Dr. Sutherland was able to delineate the subtle rhythm of this respiratory mechanism and found that its rate of three to eight cycles per minute was significantly different from the respiratory rate of twelve to fourteen breaths per minute or the heart rate of sixty to eighty beats per minute. In other words, the central nervous system, skull, spine, sacrum, and pelvis have their own ebb and flow within one's body that is unique and not the result of the breath or heart rate.

The cerebrospinal fluid drains out of the cranium through the venous blood flow that goes through a variety of sinuses (veins) throughout the cranium and brain. The dura mater that surrounds the brain provides separation within the brain as well as separation between the right and left side and the lower cerebellum from the two hemispheres above. This thick dura mater also covers the spinal cord and attaches to the coccyx and connects to various points along the spine including the sacrum, the cervical vertebrae, and the entry at the base of the skull called the foramen magnum.

When I was attending allopathic medical school, I had the opportunity to learn some basic cranial osteopathy, which I continued to train in over the years. This experience demonstrated that powerful and long-lasting healing can occur by working with this particular level of expansion and contraction in the body.

The dura mater that covers the central nervous system, including the brain, the cerebellum, and the spinal cord down to the coccyx, is intricately involved with the breath as it is acted upon through the exercises mentioned above. Perhaps then it is possible to consider that this primary respiration mechanism is mediating biochemical, electrical gradients through communication with the cerebrospinal fluid that passes through both lateral ventricles, the third and fourth ventricles, the central canal, the meninges between the cerebral hemispheres of the brain, and the dura mater that separates the cerebellum from the occipital lobe (see figure 14.2).

Many of the more sensitive regions in our nervous system, such as the vagus nuclei near the fourth ventricle and the hippocampus and the lateral ventricles, remain very close to the cerebrospinal fluid. Therefore, not only do these exercises strengthen the muscular aspects of spine to improve resiliency, they also influence the dura mater and the whole central nervous system, which assists in accessing meditative states. In

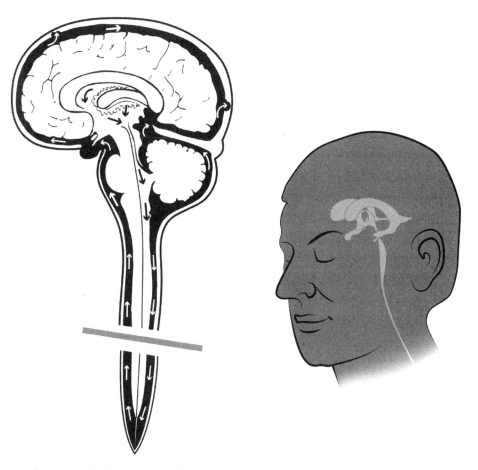

Figure 14.2. Cerebrospinal fluid path around the brain and spinal cord (left) and within the two fluid-filled lateral ventricles, third and fourth ventricles, shown in relation to the facial features (right).

fact there are many who experience kundalini and describe a path that follows the flow of the cerebrospinal fluid.

## KUNDALINI

Meditation and spiritual growth have long been identified as going hand in hand, but what may have been often overlooked is the anatomical link between them, which may be the cerebrospinal fluid that is found in the central nervous system. This fluid, the vagus nerve, and the ability to adapt and recover health are intrinsically linked with breath, and these same systems correlate to another energy system commonly discussed in yoga: kundalini.

Kriya yoga techniques when well developed and regularly practiced awaken a human's latent potential by inspiring creative energy, known as kundalini, and encouraging it to rise within the system. This potential energy source is described as residing in the general location of the sacrum. As discussed earlier, this area is referred to as the root chakra and has a grounding influence with the physical earth. It is typically dormant until one directs intention toward waking it. There is much written about the benefits and the dangers of this energy, as it can be brought out of hibernation either spontaneously or with focused meditative techniques. Sometimes spontaneous kundalini awakenings can be disruptive to one's equilibrium, and this should be taken into consideration when working with kundalini energy. If one has a grounded sense of self and proper posture with appropriate breath and psychological support, the spiritual essence of kundalini can be quickly realized and integrated. It brings with it a deep peace and great joy that fills the spaces of one's soul.

The awareness of kundalini energy can begin in childhood with dreams or out-of-body experiences even when the child does not realize they are playing within the bio-psychic (subtle) and intello-conscious (causal) fields as described in the Cycle of Synthesis. The important thing to understand is that this type of spiritual expansion is built into the human physiology. People have refined internal technologies in order to master these energies just as we have refined other aspects of our internal ability to take advantage of our communication with the world through the five senses. We discover art, music, language, and systems like science or medicine, and we discover mathematical equations to explain the quantum universe. All that is required to tap into this matrix and work with kundalini energy or human potential is within us, but we must come from a solid physical structure and breath to find the stillpoint within. Sit up straight and breathe.

Kundalini is an expression of prana, the biopsychic subtle energy, which is latent and residing at the base of spine. It awaits spiritual exultation in order to rise. It can be felt from the coccyx up to the crown and beyond, and it has the ability to waken the chakra centers. Kundalini is described as strong, lively, and infinite and intimately connected to breath, concentration, and compassion. This energy is a flow associated with the feminine, creative, Mother Earth energy rising to meet the Spirit energy of the Absolute. It may feel like a shiver up the spine, a tingling of warmth, or a sense of vibration. It can occur as a concentration around the spine and move up the body until it reaches the head. It can feel as though it pulses, filling the body and the head with pressure, joy, excitement. These experiences vary greatly and no two experiences are the same. Striving for a particular experience is counterproductive and will not prove fruitful. In this practice a "beginner's mind" is best.

In the science of tantra and yoga, libido and kundalini are considered reciprocal complementary energies. While kundalini can be described as a manifestation of joy and a unifying potential psychospiritual energy, libido tends to be a diversifying kinetic biopsychic energy. With the relative rise of libido, kundalini tends to sleep, and vice versa. They are not entirely mutually exclusive as it is a relative reciprocal relationship. Kriya and other self-regulatory techniques can lead to a shift in the relative balance between kundalini and libido in the biological, psychological, and spiritual realms. In general, kundalini is associated with the higher fields of bio-psychic and intello-conscious fields, and libido falls into the lowers fields of electro-magnetic and bio-psychic. As you can see there is overlap here and that is the nature of Nature. There are very few absolutes in the realms of normal waking consciousness.

Kundalini is an energy that is usually spoken of in conjunction with the chakras. As discussed in chapter 8, the chakras coincide roughly with various interwoven groupings of nerves near the spinal cord of the autonomic nervous system referred to as plexuses. Although there is no specific anatomical finding for any particular chakra, most individuals can identify different levels of awareness that correspond to the various chakras. For example, the heart chakra is typically felt as a place of love and compassion. We will often rub our forehead to help us think when we're trying to focus on something. The forehead corresponds to the third-eye chakra and is considered the center of true Knowledge. This is all the same energy going through the same neural pathways, but we experience it differently at different levels. Being able to transmute the same energy into different sensory phenomena depending on the level of the spinal cord is clearly part of the wonder of the human body.

The feelings and sensations that occur in a kundalini release can be intense and even become overwhelming to a practitioner who has not intended nor expected this experience. It may be mildly disorienting, but one can restore calm by returning to the breath while maintaining erect posture. However, it is more often a deeply integrating experience, especially if one is prepared with a practice that is firmly rooted in proper posture and breath.

Often kundalini release is spontaneous, but it may also be subtle and occur over many years and only be realized in hindsight. Kundalini is an expression of creation, the exultation of breath resonating within the body and the central nervous system, and the spiritual essence inside each human. With kundalini one begins to feel a greater sense of connectedness to Self. It should also be noted here that kundalini is not necessarily a one-time occurrence. While the initial presentation can sometimes be quite significant and really grabs one's attention, repeated visits with the energy become more routine and familiar and are utilized in meditation as well as other energetic practices. Kundalini teaches one about the energetic processes associated with our central nervous system and breath and with practice allows one to become adept at making the most of its presence.

Unfortunately, the concept of kundalini has often been misrepresented and taken out of context. It has become confused and entangled with notions of esoteric sexual practices related to tantra. This is a disappointing distraction from the true essence of kundalini. In fact, it is no more or less related to sex than any of our five senses. For example, although touch is certainly a part of a sexual relationship, its utility goes far beyond sexual behavior, since we also use it to accomplish many tasks in daily routine like eating, holding, driving, and sensing temperature. The experience of kundalini may influence sexual behavior but it is not a sexual practice.

It is inappropriate for teachers, mentors, and guides to present a kundalini practice as a sexual one. Doing so also creates an imbalanced power dynamic between the teacher and the student, who is openly trusting that the teacher will help lead them to true spiritual experiences. It is better for practitioners to connect to their own sense of knowing when opening to the advanced experience of kundalini. This inner knowing cannot be found in any text or taught by any master. Teachers can only lead us to the path while reminding and nurturing us to continue to seek within. Sometimes, when the situation is appropriate, a guide will also provide a not so subtle push here and there. It is clearly useful to have a trusted guide, an experienced practitioner to help you along the path, but nothing is more useful than a heartfelt, curious desire to feel the Infinite. To work with kundalini energy one must remain open and willing to become immersed with the world within, rather than approach it like a process requiring rigid direction, control, or manipulation of energy.

Kriya yoga is based on four relatively simple physiological exercises, V1–V4, that when mastered, integrated, and practiced together lead the way to physiological changes and meditative states that allow deeper levels of contemplation, prayer, self-discovery, kundalini experiences, and potential Self-Realization. You should now understand enough of the fundamentals to go forth and undertake this path with reverence and curiosity. It should not be treated frivolously, as the techniques although simple are powerful. We invite you to consider that pranayama and the power it has to transform our being is a devotional act, an acknowledgement of that interconnected relationship and sacred interdependence of the human form and what we call God, Nature, or Spirit.

# 15

# Kriya and the Practice
# of Compassion

*Be free to experience the joy of being fully present, here and
now. You will never cease to be amazed by the wonders
that there are to behold as you meander down
the royal path of Kriya yoga.*

It is early in the morning as you step outside to breathe the air. As your
lungs fill deeply, you gaze toward the sky and notice its ever-changing
nuances. Whether it is cloudy, raining, or crystal clear, the sky is always
full of pure Nature in all her glory. Breathe her in, feel her, love her,
honor her, and she will do the same for you. Compassion is the sharing
of the spirit of Nature with other sentient beings. Breathe in the joy of
the morning and take it with you throughout the day. It will provide
great solace while at the same time guide you on your way to share the
loving-kindness of breath as you make your way.

While the practice of compassion may not provide a quick fix,
reverse the immediate threat of a physical trauma, or relieve the pressure of psychological trauma immediately, it can provide a slow and
steady balancing effect on the overall health of the body, mind, and
spirit. One way it does this is by allowing the mind to become more

focused on softer and subtler energies. When one tunes in to oneself in this way there is very little chance of failure, as compassion can grow in unimaginable ways. Expanding the heart center assists one in practicing loving-kindness for oneself, and that kindness, tolerance, and reduced reactivity is extended to others as well.

There are many studies demonstrating the reduction of stress with meditative practice, breathwork, and yoga. The breath, posture, and internal focus practices of yoga can be incorporated into any faith-based practice and all walks of life. The expanded state of consciousness that one attains through focused breath and proper posture will help anyone achieve a deeper relationship with one's self and the infinite. Compassion is a heart-minded practice that guides the Spirit and the self back to one another and allows for the blossoming of the true Self in all its glory. It is ultimately our personal choice to create from a place of love rather than fear and that choice impacts all of life. This is not to say that this task is easy, but it is one well worth taking on.

Compassion is a gateway experience toward greater tolerance, expanded love, and Self-Realization that has a desired and positive effect on the body, mind, and spirit. Choosing to start with a cognitive focus on compassion and attempting to feel love for oneself, one's family, or more broadly other people in the world has a definite positive effect on one's emotional states as well as one's actions. Should the practitioner suffer from poor self-esteem, previous trauma, or self-deprecating patterns, it may be difficult for them to focus the mind on compassion. In such situations a psychotherapist may be able to assist.

If compassion feels unnatural, centering the mind around another pleasant idea is a good alternative. Watching a bee gathering pollen, the flicker of a candle, or the breeze in the trees provides ample space for the mind to rest. One can also just focus on the breath entering the heart center and feel it expand. An exquisite example of a heart opening to the cosmos is the painting of St. Francis of Assisi shown in figure 15.1 on page 230.

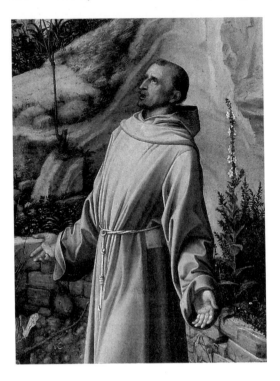

Figure 15.1. Detail from *St. Francis in the Desert,* a painting by Giovanni Bellini. This painting demonstrates an open heart chakra. The full painting currently owned by the Frick museum in New York City also demonstrates the relationship of St. Francis to the Nature and Spirit around him.

A change in posture, breathing into the heart center, and chanting can all contribute to the shift toward generating compassion toward oneself and others. This movement toward the experience of deep compassion can likely be made considerably faster using Kriya yoga techniques while at the same time remaining open to and embracing the Buddhist teachings of loving-kindness. Practicing the two together often provides greater power and more immediate results. The long-standing bhakti yoga practices, from which compassion and loving-kindness meditation sprang, hold a wealth of teachings and traditional writings to draw upon.

Having compassion is meeting suffering with love and courage. Compassion is a noun but its value is in action. Compassion is the ability to feel empathy while mobilizing action to relieve suffering. The ability to act with compassion naturally grows from the practice of Kriya. The attainment of compassion blossoms as one moves toward Self-Realization. To identify suffering in others is important and to turn compassion inward is an even more advanced technique.

The root of all compassionate actions, all spirituality, and Self-Realization is unconditional love and the ability to feel the interconnectedness of everyone and everything. It is an opportunity to bring the U3 into focus between two or more human beings in a unifying action of love. We include this here because compassion is a body-mind process that uses prana, vibration at a high level. It is a form of communication in the bio-psychic field (subtle body) that can elevate to include the cosmos as in Self-Realization, as in an experience of the intello-conscious field (causal body): God in action so to speak. In Buddhist teachings compassion is sometimes known as the "quivering of the heart" a transmutation of altruistic love, a deeply embodied courage to feel connected to oneself, others, animals, and nature. In this regard, we may consider compassion to be a form of emotional intelligence, a bio-psychic energy, a way of cultivating the inner pathway to greater acceptance, unconditional love and a deep awakening with our core.

Compassion is a delicate balance between human emotions. It is unlike empathy in that it is cultivated rather than a learned behavior. Empathy is described as the embodied feeling of another person's pain and suffering. The unfortunate side of empathy is the possibility of becoming burned out by being empathetic. Many can easily feel someone else's emotional experience but are unable to move past it or let go of it. Empathy without actionable compassion can contribute to burnout, fatigue, and cognitive distortions creating resentment and anger. One cannot have empathy for oneself in the same way one can have compassion, and compassion engenders a healthy detachment while mobilizing action. Practicing compassion is another way to promote self-care and awareness of one's boundaries.

As French Buddhist monk Matthieu Ricard once said, "When altruistic love passes through the prism of empathy, it becomes compassion." Compassion is in fact the art of love and loving without distraction or attachment to outcome. It allows for and engenders a healthy detachment while mobilizing action.

Imagine that compassion has a density, a texture, a color that you can interact with, and as you practice holding compassion at the forefront of your mind's eye and heart, you will find a seed of acceptance within yourself and the ability to cultivate it every day. Such an exercise has the potential to shift the physiological reactions in the body and mind and practicing and embodying these experiences will bring about long-lasting neuroplastic changes. Compassion is arguably one of the most valuable gifts we have as humans. It has the power to remove suffering and its cause.

## ≪ Compassion Exercise

Sit bolt upright paying attention to the spine and maintaining it as a column of structure and energy. Be in your spine, feel the strength in your ability to sit and elongate your back. The goal is to find a neutral balance in the spinal curves.

Imagine your spine is like a tree reaching deep into the earth and up into the sky and feel it gently tethered between the two poles. Remain flexible, supple, and relaxed. Feel solid and balanced and ready to act. Drop your awareness into your pelvis (use a pillow for extra support if needed) and send your tailbone into the earth for a grounding influence. Allow both sit bones to balance the weight of your body with gravity. Allow the lumbar curve to hold your frame while avoiding overflattening or overbending this part of your back.

Allow your hands to rest on your thighs, knees, or lap. Intentionally relax your shoulders, squeezing the shoulder blades gently back and together to decrease the space between them and pressing the shoulders gently away from the ears, while simultaneously allowing the sternum to lift with the breath. The lower area of the sternum is where most people experience the heart chakra emanating its energy, and this where we will focus with compassion meditation.

Gently lift the back of the head, elongating your cervical spine, and shift your forehead forward and down while allowing your chin to drop slightly toward the chest. With these motions the back portion of the top of your head, the vertex, moves closer to the sky. The neck should be long without much curving at the shoulders. Tucking the chin down creates a slight pressure in the thyroid/throat area, which assists in breath and prana control. The mouth is relaxed with a slight smile, the eyebrows are raised, and the tongue is touching the palate of your mouth behind the front teeth. The eyes may be open with a unfocused gaze at a 45 degree angle toward the floor, closed gently, or closed while gazing toward the space between the eyebrows, the third eye/gyral center, without strain.

Once this position is achieved return your awareness to the the sternum, your heart center, and breathe into that spot for a moment. Now hold it for a moment. Play with the feeling of further expansion and try to generate a whole-body sense of compassion about something or someone. Imagine the channels of energy in the body coming awake and tune in to sensations within while also tuning in to your antenna. The goal is to align your nervous system/physiology with your energy body as well as with Spirit. This is an embodied experience and should be felt in a very real physical sense.

Continue with mindful breath becoming more aligned with the essence of breath, feeling each cell and imagining it being bathed in Spirit. As the center of the chest grows warm, expand it out bit by bit with each inhalation and with each slow exhalation be mindful to maintain the sternum high and not let the chest collapse. Slowly breathe into the expansion of the heart and a peaceful silence. Follow the breath into the deepest regions of the heart. Imagine the heart center glowing with an internal warmth that begins to permeate the skin. This light begins to melt the frozen areas of the heart, opening it up to have more compassion for what the body has endured, softening to the human experience and its universality.

Take this exercise as slowly as you need to, focusing on the unhurried, subtle expansion of the heart center. Hold this image in your mind and imagine that its light and warmth grow to fill every crevice of the body, every corner of the heart until there is only light radiating to fill the space around you.

By learning to embody compassion in conjunction with Kriya breath one gains the ability to fully embrace the embodiment of altruistic love and compassion at a moment's notice by slightly shifting to an awareness of the breath while activating a mindful heart.

Developing compassion for self and others can greatly accelerate one's growth. Any faith one may practice can only benefit from understanding that this devotional act is a prayer in itself, a prostration to a higher force and an honoring of self and the force within.

*There is no religion higher than Truth, and there is no Truth higher than Compassion.*
ROXANNE, KAMAYANI GUPTA,
*THE YOGA OF INDIAN CLASSICAL DANCE*

# Final Thoughts on the Teachings of Kriya

*Love, Love, Love.*

PARAMAHAMSA PRAJNANANANDA

*Have patience and do your practice systematically.*
*This is the secret to a successful practice.*

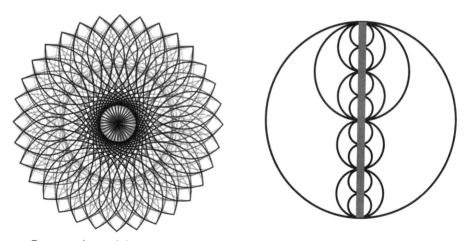

Two visual mandala representations of infinity. (Circular drawing on right by Eve Neuhaus from her book *The Crazy Wisdom of Ganesh Baba.*) The Sri Yantra (see figure 2.1 on page 29) and the Cycle of Synthesis (see figure 5.1 on page 60) are further attempts to describe the infinite experience of U3.

All in all, Kriya yoga is a process of individualized creative integration of the body, mind, and spirit. It is a series of exercises that have been practiced for hundreds and likely thousands of years with subtle variations. It is both an art and a science and sits squarely at the base of all the contemplative arts and religions. It requires no belief system and does not suggest anybody alter the current devotional practices or change their religion in order to practice Kriya. Kriya yoga provides a highly structured and stable path with which to explore the psychospiritual realms of human development and evolution.

The teachings of Kriya yoga are for everyone. Kriya, just like all other self-regulatory techniques, belongs to everyone. Ganesh Baba taught Kriya yoga as an open source software that could be downloaded by any "human biocomputer," a term that he was fond of using. It was his goal to share his knowledge and experience with anyone who was interested. Of course, like any field of study, it takes time, effort, and dedication to learn and become proficient in it, and there are not many who choose to put in that effort.

As one approaches a new field of study such as Kriya, or any other subject for that matter, it is helpful to have an overview of the path ahead in a clear, simple but complete fashion so that one can understand the course of study as they move through it. Self-regulatory techniques are no different, and the purpose of this book is to outline the basic foundational steps for Kriya yoga meditation in a comprehensive, yet approachable manner. It is also an attempt to honor Ganesh Baba's dedication to teaching others and continuing the trail of footprints from the teachers that came before him.

That said, one has to be patient in both teaching and learning Kriya yoga. It takes time to become proficient in the basic techniques, let alone the more advanced ones. As with many self-regulatory practices the advanced details become apparent to the practitioner as they move along on the path and reach the appropriate level of understanding to continue to move forward. It is not uncommon for advanced techniques to all of a sudden become available to the practitioner through a fellow traveler, a teacher whose path they cross, or one's inner guide. As stated earlier, the true teacher is within and any physical teacher with whom one has contact is there only to help prepare the groundwork and potentially provide a little push to help one take the first steps down the path. As with a toddler learning to walk, the initial steps can be quite challenging and having someone around to provide support and direction can be very helpful. However, history is full of examples of those who found the path and made their way along it without a clear map or guide.

If anything, Kriya yoga teaches that everything you need, you already have, but it also provides direction and support as the Kriya network is broad and interconnected in ways that defy the rational mind's idea of cause and effect. Kriya yoga provides direct experience with the concept of synchronicity, the acausal connecting principle, that brings coincidence without direct causation into one's daily life. This does not mean that hardship is removed, but one's resiliency is certainly increased by having a more robust nervous system and increasing one's deep knowledge of impermanence and detachment. This by itself decreases much of what the Buddhists refer to as suffering. Truly living in the moment with a sense of impermanence and detachment provides new levels of human experience.

Modern day Kriya yoga as taught in its recent incarnation in the Kriya lineage of Lahiri Mahasaya stresses that Kriya should stay a householder practice. Lahiri believed that if Kriya was practiced by teachers, cooks, farmers, weavers, and scientists, it could change society. There are accounts of him stating that ashrams and organizations should not develop around Kriya, as they would inherently involve politics and human nature, which would have a negative impact on Kriya's transmission from generation to generation. As one looks around at the various ways to learn Kriya, it is clear that many of Lahiri's disciples did in fact begin schools that then became institutions in their own right. Some remain alive and full of love, inspiration, and activity. Unfortunately, others have become somewhat rigid and brittle. That is not to say that those that have aged less well than others cannot be reinvigorated, as the essence of Kriya is there only waiting to be awakened again.

Once one experiences the power of Kriya yoga or has success with other self-regulatory techniques, one cannot simply walk away and pretend it never happened. Peoples' perceptions are changed to such a degree that they cannot return to the previous way they viewed the universe. For example, as one progresses deeper into these self-regulatory techniques, their experiences can lead to perceptions of time that are markedly different from what they have imagined. The Cycle of Synthesis provides some insight into how that can be conceptualized.

Direct experience of the cosmos beyond time shifts one's concept of "reality" in a radical way. Time is a concept that we use to measure movement in relation to our experience of life. Through Kriya and other techniques it can become apparent that time does not exist in the same way we are used to experiencing it. As shown in the Cycle of Synthesis, there are energies that move beyond time but yet still exist.

These concepts have been written about in ancient scriptures and in particular within the rich tradition of Vedanta. The same ideas are now being measured by physicists as they increasingly delve into previously hidden secrets of black holes. One way to think of the universe beyond time is to use the idea of a hologram. A hologram is when a three-dimensional image is captured on a film such that any single spot on the hologram contains all the information needed to reconstruct the whole image. Now try and imagine a four-dimensional hologram. Such a hologram would contain all the time that there ever was and ever will be. In a sense this would be a holographic picture of infinity. This exercise in imagination begins to give one an idea of the reality that is beyond the four-dimensional space-time continuum that we know so well.

We move forward in our lives as time moves past in the opposite direction in the fourth dimensional space-time continuum. We cannot slow time down, budget it, pace it, or save it. Time is not something we can "accumulate." None of the relationships, feelings, or things we have will move on with us when our physical life ends, and our time is up in this realm. The only thing that will continue on is our soul.

Perhaps we might be humbled to consider ourselves stewards of life and our time in it. How might we manage our resources while we are alive in the most respectful way for others and for the planet? For many spiritual pursuits, the goal is to reach "enlightenment" and spend one's time there and often away from society as a whole. The opposite is true in Kriya yoga where if one does experience levels of Self-Realization, one's goal is to bring that Realization right back into one's life as a householder and move forward with the work in front of them.

When experiencing levels of Self-Realization it becomes inherently clear that the scriptures are in fact correct and that there is no ultimate separation in any aspect of our experience. Kriya yoga masters speak about a conscious, volitional death, referred to as mahasamadhi, that occurs in Kriya yoga when one takes one's last breath. It is believed in many Eastern societies that if one reaches that level of breath control within one's lifetime then there is some choice as to whether to return for another reincarnation in this fourth dimensional space-time continuum. "Some things in life have to be seen to be believed" and in this case they have to be experienced. Do not doubt the power of Kriya yoga.

In the expanding physical universe time is not infinite, but a reservoir of the future for the fourth dimensional space-time continuum so to speak. From our human perspective we spend time with little thought, using terse phrases like "what a waste of time" or "how to pass the time" or "killing time." What exactly is a waste of time? Our life is comprised of moments, and it is something we can share as long as we are still, to quote Swami Hariharananda, "pulling breath." It is the ultimate Spirit of the universe that sparks our breath, is it not? It is only the Absolute that is beyond time that brings life to the physical universe.

Toward the end of his life Sri Yukteswar is described as being irritated one day by those around him when they wanted him to bathe. He responded, "There is no time for that" and went on to say that he wanted to spend his remaining time in meditation. Each breath is a measure of time. How is it that you will utilize this resource? If each breath can be taken in full, relaxed reposed fashion with straight posture your relationship with time will be transformed both in the here and now and with the Infinite. Kriya yoga is one such technique that if utilized on a regular basis can help an individual gain insight into the nature of reality that is beyond duality and is the U3.

## THE ART OF THE PRACTICE

The Practice of Kriya yoga helps us integrate our internal experience of expanded awareness with that of the world around us. We may progress beyond imagined limitations and accept life as it happens, engage in the moments in which we find ourselves, and feel joy in the space between choice and action. Mastering the skills of concentration and guided breath assists us in mastering our attention. With this we can choose our experiences. We may not have control over the weather or the traffic, but we can develop the gift of altruistic love.

As we allow compassionate contemplation to occur, it sinks deeper within and permeates the whole of our lives. Meditate on loving-kindness, acceptance, and the gifts of Nature and act with altruistic intention. This brings synchronicity into alignment with the life one leads. The practitioner of Kriya will soon realize the body and mind, spirit and emotion in new ways.

When we learn to do this through meditation, we attain the highest of all joys that can ever be experienced by a human being. All the other joys in the world are momentary, but the joy of meditation is immense and everlasting. This is not an exaggeration; it is a truth supported by the long line of sages; those who renounced the world and attained Truth, and those who continued living in the world yet remained unaffected by it. Meditation teaches you to systematically explore your inner dimensions. It is a system of commitment and of creative communion, not commandment. You are committing to yourself, to your path, and to the goal of knowing yourself. While learning to be calm and still need not be a ceremony or religious ritual, it is a universal requirement for the evolution of the human body, mind, and spirit.

## *Cultivating Stillness*

Learning how to be still is a state that is experienced through practicing the various methods of meditation. The process of cultivating stillness begins with the body and meditation and becomes no more difficult than putting on your shoes before leaving the house in the morning. In the yoga tradition, you are guided by a competent teacher to keep your head, neck, and trunk straight while sitting in a meditative posture (asana). When you have learned to be comfortable in this posture, you should form a regular habit of practicing in the same posture at the same time and at the same place every day. You may become very aware of how thoughts make you feel, how feelings can cause reactivity, and how restless the mind is. It tosses and turns like you do on a night when you cannot fall asleep. But that is only a problem when you identify with the mind and react to the various thoughts it throws at you. If you do react, you will be caught in a never-ending whirlwind of restless activity, for it is not the thoughts that disturb you, it's your reaction to them.

*It is all in the breath!*

This is the time to return to the breath, for it is the breath that controls the mind. If thoughts abound simply return to the breath, attend to those thoughts with compassion as they arise, without reacting, or if you react then attend to the reaction. In this way these thoughts cannot really disturb you. In fact they can be considered gentle reminders to stay focused on V1–V4, for the breath smooths out a sea of confusion by calming the waters.

So begin by attending to your breath. Meditation teaches you to attend to what is taking place within without reacting. It brings you freedom from the mind and its meandering and in this freedom you begin to experience who you are, distinct from your mental turmoil.

You experience inner joy and contentment, you experience relief and inner relaxation, and you find a respite from the tumultuousness of your life. You have given yourself an inner vacation while at the same time allowing for growth and integration. This inner vacation is not a retreat from the world but the foundation for finding inner peace and getting to know yourself. You must also learn to apply the principle of attending to your worldly activities, so that you can function in the world more effectively. Through practicing compassionate meditation, you can learn to be open to what comes and give it your full attention.

## Working with a Teacher

Although first and foremost, it is best to begin with one's own inner teacher, it may be beneficial to consider working with an outside teacher who will gently challenge you to push yourself while helping you remain flexible and safe. Any inwardly focused work can activate anxiety as an individual moves through emotions, memories, and traumas that have been held within the body. Sometimes these old traumas float to the surface as grief or sadness, and while this can be the beginning of an integrative process, it can still be unsettling. The support of a counselor or therapist well-versed in self-regulatory techniques can be a helpful aid if one has a history of trauma, depression, or anxiety.

There are also some situations where engaging in these practices should not occur at all unless one is supervised by a physician or psychologist. This includes anyone that has previously experienced any type of psychotic disorder. Anyone experiencing episodes of dissociation may also want to consult with a psychiatrist or psychologist before moving forward with self-regulatory techniques, particularly if they are practicing alone. In addition, some of the more aggressive pranayama techniques are not indicated in individuals who are pregnant or have difficulties with hypertension or heart disease.

There is no question that spiritual awakenings happen spontaneously as many religions have formed around such occurrences, but a guide or teacher can help manage these symptoms and situations in a proper and health-promoting way. Historically, it was common for someone on a spiritual path to find a teacher and live with that teacher in some way for a period of time, typically years. Sometimes these relationships were in a monastery or ashram-like setting but more often than not they were individual relationships. In the West the ability to go and live with the teacher is fairly limited. However, the more contact one has with a teacher, the more information can be transferred. A teacher's true task is to pull the truth from within the student and reflect it most honestly.

Remember also that it is not just the student who finds the teacher, but also the teacher that finds the student. Teachers and so-called gurus are many while true students are few. It has been said that one step by a student is often met with ten steps by the teacher. However, blind trust is not appropriate. Teachers are human, too, with strengths and weaknesses, perspectives, opinions, and beliefs. For this reason, it is best not to move too quickly between teachers, for while it might make the practice interesting and full of flavor, it will not provide the most benefit or help to refine one's skills.

As one proceeds along the spiritual development path, one's energy/vibration changes. This is important to understand when seeking out a teacher, as a teacher should have reached a point where the inter- and intrapersonal precepts have become embodied. The demands of practice can impact a student in profound ways, and it is always helpful to have a trusted advisor to assist in moments of confusion, but a student leading a student is like the blind leading the blind. This not a good path as it potentially adds to many wrong turns if relative beginners are going down a bumpy road in the dark. When one chooses to follow a path, it should be chosen with consideration to the physical, biological, psychological, and the spiritual aspects of knowledge. To develop a good working relationship that provides steady growth, each of these levels must resonate with the student and the teacher. Both teacher and student will flip between guide and guided over the course of this journey. There is no competent teacher that is not first and foremost a curious and active student at every moment, especially when teaching.

## Signs of Progress

Every action has a reaction. It is not possible for you to meditate and not receive benefits. You may not notice those benefits right away; however, your nervous system is having new experiences that promote integration and growth. These neuroplastic changes will settle deep within and be there for you later. If you sow a seed today, you won't reap the fruit tomorrow, but eventually you will have a tree full of ripe delicious fruit full of seeds for more trees.

It takes time to see results; be gentle but firm and honest with yourself. Meditation means carefully fathoming all the levels of your being, one after another. When working with the mind, you need patience. You need to develop a cooperative working relationship with yourself, your posture, and your breath to influence the mind. Learn to love your breath, and it will love you and assist you on this path.

Some of the most important benefits of meditation make themselves known over time in subtle ways and are not dramatic or easily observed. At first you may see progress in terms of physical relaxation and emotional calmness. Later you may notice other changes. Persist in your practice, and you will find that meditation is a means of freeing yourself from the worries that gnaw at you. Then you can experience the joy of being fully present, here and now. You will never cease to be amazed by the wonders there are to behold as you meander down the royal path of Kriya yoga.

## IN CLOSING

*With proper posture comes a straight back and straight breath.*
GANESH BABA

We are now at the end of this particular journey. If you have been inspired, you have already begun to embrace some of the practices described in this book. From this point on it is practice, practice, practice at the same time and in the same place every day and preferably twice a day. This is the way to achieve accelerated progress. That said, any amount of practice is beneficial, although a small amount of practice every day is much more beneficial than longer duration practices that are not daily.

As we are coming to a close, there are a couple more points to get across regarding practice. As mentioned, association is very important. Practicing at the same time of day in the same space adds additional power to the practice. In addition is it said that facing north or east is best. Please remember that it is the frequency of practice that is much more important than the length of time one practices for. Someone who puts forth daily effort for even five minutes will progress much faster than one who puts in a two hour session once a week. That said, there is a natural quieting in the central nervous system that happens after fifteen to twenty minutes. When possible, daily practice for this amount of time with longer sessions on occasion will provide the structure for someone who is determined to move forward at a quicker pace.

What you've read here is a roadmap to the hardware and software that you already have within you. There is no secret passage that you need to find. You just need to spend time sitting and breathing and know that it is not possible to engage in these tasks and not have a shift in your conscious awareness and experience of being human. Although we have covered many details in this book, the most important ones are, of course, having a straight back and proceeding with a straight breath. If that is all you do, the rest will still come in time. Enjoy the journey, and as Longfellow said and Ganesh Baba often repeated as the essence of Kriya yoga . . .

> *Trust no Future, howe'er pleasant!*
> *Let the dead Past bury its dead!*
> *Act,—act in the living Present!*
> *Heart within, and God o'erhead!*
> EXCERPT FROM "A PSALM OF LIFE"
> BY HENRY WADSWORTH LONGFELLOW

Grace alone is in charge from this point forward. May these writings find those who may be looking for them, and may the blessings of the breath bring joy on your journey and to those whose paths you cross.

\* \* \*

Namaste

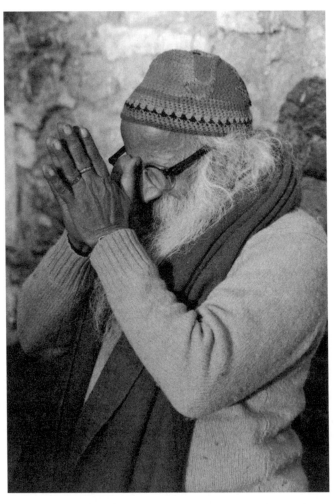

Ganesh Baba in France, in 1986 or 1987.
(Photo by Michelle Cruzel.)

APPENDIX I

# Nature, Psychedelics, and Meditation

Botanical and medical anthropology has informed us that humans have engaged in various methods of altering consciousness for millennia. In fact, it may have been the accidental ingestion of psychoactive plant material that contributed to the dawn of ancient religious practices. As time progressed, it became evident to some that similar transcendental experiences could be experienced through the human body without the aid of an exogenous substance. In some areas, such as India, both schools of thought coexist, although it should be noted that psychoactive substances are not used by traditional healers, shamans, yogis, or nagas for entertainment or distraction. In fact, psychoactive plant material is considered sacred and is used only at certain times and situations with specific expectations and rules of engagement.

In the past few hundred years there has been an increase in crosscultural exchange, and a variety of sacred rituals from various cultures across the globe have become games of distraction and euphoria for westerners. Most notable in this group in the West were the hippies of the 1960s and '70s.

Some saw the rise of the hippie movement as degenerative and amoral, and others saw the potential of seeing our world in a new way, or

247

should I say an old way, where humans are really one with the environment, and destruction of the environment is no different from engaging in self-harm. Unfortunately, the "free love" aspect of the hippie movement that was associated with "sex, drugs, and rock 'n' roll" was unable to maintain the inherent focus expressed in the saying "all you need is love" and moved instead to a more hedonistic approach of sensory pleasures. That said, however, the movement did ultimately leave some new ideas and initial changes behind, but they were subsequently squelched by inertia as the 1980s began.

What we were left with is a culture that was more accepting of a freer sexuality, which led to a media obsession with appearance, attraction, and sexuality with little to no focus on the development of the heartfelt aspects of compassion. From a substance-use standpoint, the psychedelics that were used at the time, including cannabis in its various forms, LSD, peyote, psilocybin, and others, were used as entertainment, and their use as a sacrament was largely ignored. Although many individuals experienced a marked change in their worldview through the use of psychedelic substances, there was no underlying structure or ability within most individuals to carry that with them throughout their life to inform their relationships with themselves or others.

One aspect of the psychedelic experience was increased awareness of nature. And although the environmental movement began at that time and continued with some force, small gains were accepted as evidence of progress and positive change within Western countries with little understanding of the massive global raping of the planet's precious natural resources. And as developing countries moved more toward a Western style of consumption, developed nations sat happy and intoxicated with the small successes that occurred.

Although some have written about Ganesh Baba's relationships with psychedelics, he was first and foremost against their use in anyone who had not yet reached retirement age. Of course, he had no control of those around him and despite discouraging psychedelic use among young people, including the casual use of marijuana, he would strongly enforce his doctrine of straight back and straight breath if one was using a psychedelic substance.

The same goes for young marijuana users today. If they wish to continue using marijuana and do not want to stop even though they understand the physical and psychological risks, then I would say that any time they are in an altered state of consciousness from marijuana their back should be perfectly straight and meditation should be the task at hand. Slouched posture, shallow breathing, watching television, gossiping, staring at the ceiling, and mindlessly listening to music are all activities to avoid if one has taken a substance that has induced an altered state. Straight posture and straight breath and ideally visualization and other meditative techniques are the best use of those altered states.

From a spiritual standpoint, Ganesh Baba saw the hippie movement as an indication of the collective increase in conscious awareness in that there was more acceptance and an attempt to be more open and loving and explore other dimensions of what it means to be human. Unfortunately, his ultimate conclusion was that the rapid drug and alcohol use in those decades left many burned out and unmotivated. Many moved forward into a life working for multinational corporations, and others "dropped out," following Timothy Leary's recommendation for psychedelic users. Unfortunately, neither of those paths helped to move a true shift in human consciousness forward to where "free love" is understood as altruistic love and compassion, and psychoactive plants/ entheogens are tools for learning and insight that are not to be used and abused for hedonistic pleasures. So although there was a promising path at the time toward enlightened awareness, altruistic love, and respect for Mother Earth and other cultures, the hippies took their eye off the ball. Were they just too stoned?

I bring this topic up in this book because as of this writing in 2019, the movement for the recreational use of marijuana is prominent across North America. Are marijuana and other psychedelics evil drugs? Of course not. Psychedelics are not opiates, speed, alcohol, or tobacco. They do not belong to a class of drugs that are abused in the same fashion, although marijuana used on a regular basis clearly seems to have negative effects on a developing brain and can aggravate learning difficulties, sleep disorders, anxiety, and depression and even activate latent psychotic disorders. Certainly, the risks of psychedelics are there if individuals are not prepared beforehand.

In recent years, research for psilocybin has been taking place in medical research facilities in the West. This is certainly a welcome development, and initial studies are showing significant promise in treating some very challenging psychiatric disorders such as PTSD and severe substance abuse. There is also a movement in some areas to have psilocybin available for use among the population with few if any restrictions. This is in response to what appears to be an increasing number of individuals seeking psychedelic experiences as a way to pursue insight and inner awakenings.

Although this is not necessarily a bad thing in general, it remains highly illegal as any psychoactive substance is considered a Schedule 1 controlled substance in the United States and in many countries of the world due to international treaties in 1961 and 1971. This places psychedelics in the same category as heroin and cocaine and although the dangers of use are not similar in any way, the legal ramifications of possession or use remain severe. Despite the legal issues, the most concerning aspect of the current rise in psychedelic use is the lack of deeply trained professionals to assist those to integrate that experience. Although people do not die acutely of an overdose (but can from an accident) such as with opiates, or from a heart attack or seizure from cocaine use, some still have terrific difficulties integrating their experience after what is referred to as their "journey."

Although the focus of this book is on spirituality and not on drug use, the two can often be confused in certain situations. The point of this section is to say that the posture and breathing exercises described in this book as Kriya yoga should be considered a basic skill of anyone before they move into any type of experiment with marijuana and/ or other psychedelics. These substances all have the ability to change consciousness, which can be a blissful but also a horrific and terrifying experience. Regardless of whether or not one has a so-called "guide" with them for their "journey," the aftermath of integrated experience is the more important piece. Without skilled experts to help an individual in that realm, ongoing depression, terror, and dissociation as well as PTSD can go on for years. Some in favor of the free use of psychedelics may feel that this is an extreme warning, but having grown up in the 1960s and '70s and having worked in psychiatric settings since the 1980s, I have personally seen almost every experience imaginable. It is with that background that I put forward the caution here given the rapid change in use patterns that is currently going on in North America. That said, nothing in the statements above should be construed as endorsement of harsh criminal penalties for substances that have no evidence of showing addictive properties. It is very clear that alcohol and tobacco, both freely available in shops on any street corner around the world, are markedly more destructive to human health, relationships, and the rising cost of medical care than the group of psychedelic plants loosely referred to as entheogens.

# APPENDIX II
# Additional Resources

The lists below contain the names of organizations and titles of videos that might be helpful on your Kriya yoga path. Some are Kriya yoga specific, and others are related to mindfulness and meditation. All of them have value; you'll have to see which ones resonate with you. For additional information regarding Kriya yoga as presented in this book go to **https://KriyaBreath.com**.

## ORGANIZATIONS

Not everyone who claims to teach Kriya has experience with a master and that clearly limits transmission of the essence of Kriya. Be wise and trust your inner guide as you move forward. That said, there are clearly realized souls in all of the organizations below, although those individuals are not always readily available to people who come knocking on the door. Remember: a teacher should be compassionate, loving, and generous in all ways. If a facility or individual does not feel like a good fit, try another.

- Le Centre de Yoga Tripoura—Christian Pilastre was made Kriya acharya (instructor) by Ganesh Baba in 1980. He is also a yoga teacher in the Sivananda line. He and his wife, Martine, run this center, which is in the west of France.
- Benson-Henry Institute for Mind Body Medicine at Massachusetts

General Hospital—151 Merrimac Street, 4th Floor, Boston, Mass. 02114. Programs, professional training, and referrals.
- The UMass Memorial Health Care Center for Mindfulness, 365 Plantation Street, Worcester, Mass. 01605. Professional training and referrals.
- The Center for Mind-Body Medicine, 5225 Connecticut Avenue, NW, Washington, D.C. 20015. Programs, professional training, and referrals.
- Transcendental Meditation, Maharishi International University, Fairfield, Iowa 52556. Transcendental meditation programs, training, and referrals.
- Self-Realization Fellowship, 3880 San Rafael Avenue, Los Angeles, Calif. 90065. Kriya yoga formed by Paramahansa Yogananda.
- Kriya Yoga Institute, P.O. Box 924615, Homestead, Fla. 33092-4615. Kriya Yoga instruction by Paramahamsa Prajnanananda principle disciple of Paramahamsa Hariharananda who was disciple of Sri Yukteswar.
- Rajahamsa Swami Nityananda Giri, Lakshman Jhula, Rishikesh, disciple of Paramahamsa Hariharananda. See Rajahamsa Kriya and Nityananda Giri Kriya Yoga websites.
- Center for Spiritual Awareness, P.O. Box 7, Lakemont, Georgia 30552. Founded by Roy Eugene Davis, a disciple of Paramahansa Yogananda.
- Center for Spiritual Enlightenment, 1146 University Avenue, San Jose, Calif., 95126. Founded by Yogacharya Ellen Grace O'Brian, a disciple of Roy Eugene Davis.
- Sri Rangin Mukherjee. See Original Kriya website. From the Lineage of Lahiri Mahasaya through Swami Pranabananda Giri and Shri Gyanendranath Mukhopadhyay.
- Himalayan Yoga Tradition (HYT), The Meditation Center, 631 University Avenue N.E., Minneapolis, Minn. 55413 or AHYMSIN, 744 Goldenroad Street, Escondido, Calif. 92027.
- The Bihar School of Yoga, Ganga Darshan, Fort Munger, Bihar

811201, India. Founded in 1964 by Sri Swami Satyananda Saraswati.

- Ananda Village, 14618 Tyler Foote Road, Nevada City, California, 95959. Founded by Swami Kriyananda, a disciple of Paramahansa Yogananda.
- Yoga Niketan. See website of the same name.

## ONLINE VIDEOS FOR PRANAYAMA

There are many online videos about pranayama. The following sites have authentic pranayama exercises. Look at some videos and get a general idea of what good pranayama looks like.

- Kapalbhati Step by Step Explanation by Michaël Bijker at YogaLap on YouTube
- Pranayama videos by Kavita Maharaj are very good. They are available on YouTube. Kavita runs Red Door Yoga in British Columbia.

# Chai Recipe

With Ganesh Baba, hot fresh chai was routine. He liked to drink chai all throughout the day and evening. Learning how to prepare chai to his liking was a skill quickly developed by those around him. While there are as many chai recipe variations as there are villages in India, a few standards are ubiquitous. The common ingredients are a nice strong black tea, cardamom, ginger, water, sugar, and milk. During the years I spent with Ganesh Baba he requested the addition of fennel, cinnamon, black pepper, and cloves. Occasionally I add star anise.

A mortar and pestle will be needed. Don't hesitate to adjust the proportions of the recipe to your liking. These days there are all kinds of instant versions available, but none compare to pot-made chai whose fresh ingredients fill the house with its aroma.

### Ganesh Baba's Chai Tea

*Ingredients*

5 quarter-size slices fresh ginger

1–2 cinnamon sticks

4 whole cloves

1 to 1½ tablespoons fennel seeds (crushed but not powdered)

Black peppercorns (to taste)

½ to 1 tablespoon of cardamom seeds (decorticated pods or enough whole pods from which to obtain the same amount)

1–3 star anise (optional)

Black tea of your choice. Use bulk tea or add multiple tea bags to
the pot of chai. We used Darjeeling and Earl Grey, but most
often the Lipton Yellow Label usually found at Indian food
stores. (The Lipton Yellow Label tea sold in the average U.S. gro-
cery store is not the same product.) This particular tea's unique
processing curls the leaves while they dry.

Milk or milk substitute (to taste)

Sugar or alternative sweetener (to taste)

*Process*

Add 1 quart of water to a 2-quart saucepan and place on the stove
to boil.

While water is heating, prepare and add each of the spices:

Cut 5 quarter-size slices of ginger and add to pot.

Add approximately 4 whole cloves.

Add 1–2 cinnamon sticks slightly broken open by mortar and pestle.

Add 1 to 1½ tablespoons of crushed but not powdered fennel seeds.

Freshly ground black pepper to taste.

Cardamom has a few options. With decorticated seeds, add ½ to 1
tablespoon to the mortar and pestle and grind down so that most of the
small seeds begin to crumble. If you use the whole pods, crack the shells
fairly aggressively with the mortar and pestle, at which point you can
separate the shells (time consuming) from the seeds inside or continue
to grinding the mixture until the tiny seeds begin to crumble. You can
add the shells and seeds to the water as the mixture will be strained
before drinking.

Add 1–3 star anise that have been broken open in the mortar and
pestle (optional).

And of course, the fresher the ingredients the more flavorful the
chai!

Once all the above ingredients have been added, simmer the water
for 5 to 15 minutes. Have the milk and tea ready by the stove. Add the
tea and quickly thereafter, add the milk. Boiling the tea too long can

make it bitter. Adding the milk right after adding the tea stops the boiling process. The next step is to bring the chai to a boil without letting it spill over and leave a big mess. Of course, the chai never boiled over in our house!

*A note about the milk.* You can use either whole milk or fat free milk depending on your taste. The chai can be mostly milk if you start with less water, or can be mostly water with the addition of only 10 to 25 percent milk at the end. The more milk the richer the taste. Of course, you can always try and use a nondairy alternative milk, like soy, almond, or oat although the texture can vary if boiled.

Bring the chai to the point of just boiling, and then turn it off. Repeat bringing the tea to a simmer and down again a few times to complete the process. Allow the tea to sit and steep for a couple of minutes.

Strain the chai using a ladle and a small strainer for each cup. Add sugar or another sweetener individually to taste. A little bit of sugar can go a long way to bring out the flavor of the chai. The mixture of spices at the bottom can often be reused with a little extra spice for a second or third pot if so desired.

Now sit down and enjoy while you sit straight and breathe.

# Notes

## INTRODUCTION.
## WELCOME TO THE KRIYA PATH

1. Shree Shree Anandamayee Sangha, *Mother, as Seen by Her Devotees* (1995), 39.

## 1. MEDITATION

1. Walpola Rahula, *What the Buddha Taught: Revised and Expanded Edition with Texts from Suttas and Dhammapada* (New York: Grove Atlantic, 1974).

## 2. ROOTS AND FUNDAMENTALS OF KRIYA YOGA

1. *Living in the Light: The Words and Wisdom of Paramahamsa Hariharananda,* Kriya Yoga Institute, 2006, CD.

## 3. SPIRIT-INFUSED SCIENCE

1. Walter Sullivan, "The Einstein Papers: A Man of Many Parts," *New York Times,* March 29, 1972.
2. As quoted in Dennis Overbye, "Messenger at the Gates of Time" *Science 81* 2, no. 5 (June): 66–67.
3. Wikipedia, s.v., "Bell's theorem," accessed December 22, 2019.
4. John Muir, *My First Summer in the Sierra* (Boston: Houghton Mifflin, 1911). (The quote can be found on page 110 of the Sierra Club Books 1988 edition.)

5. Albert Einstein, *Ideas and Opinions* (New York: Bonzana Books, 1954), 8–11.

## 6. SPINE BOLT UPRIGHT

1. *Awake: The Life of Yogananda* (Los Angeles: Self-Realization Fellowship, 2015), 83.

## 7. PRANAYAMA AND THE CULTIVATION OF JOY

1. *What Is Kriya Yoga?*, Paramahamsa Hariharananda Interview, 1985, YouTube video.

## 8. REFINING THE TECHNIQUES AND CREATING A KRIYA YOGA SESSION

1. Eve Neuhaus, *The Crazy Wisdom of Ganesh Baba* (Rochester, Vt.: Inner Traditions, 2010), 58.
2. Yogananda Paramahamsa, *Autobiography of a Yogi,* 6th edition (Los Angeles: Self-Realization Fellowship, 1955), 175.
3. S. W. Lazar, et al. "Meditation Experience Is Associated with Increased Cortical Thickness," *NeuroReport* 16 (2005): 1893–1897.

## 9. WELLNESS, STRESS, PSYCHOLOGY, AND KRIYA YOGA

1. Richard P. Brown and Patricia L. Gerberg, "Sudarshan Kriya Yogic Breathing in the Treatment of Stress, Anxiety, and Depression: Part I–Neurophysiologic Model," *Journal of Alternative and Complementary Medicine* 11, no. 1 (February, 2005): 189–201.
2. Gerald Murphy, *The Constitution of the Iroquois Nations: The Great Law of Peace,* EngageNY (website), December 27, 2019.

## 10. KRIYA YOGA, THE AUTONOMIC NERVOUS SYSTEM, AND THE DEVELOPMENT OF RESILIENCY

1. Keith Lowenstein, "Meditation and Self-Regulatory Techniques," in *Handbook of Complementary and Alternative Therapies in Mental Health,* edited by Scott Shannon (Cambridge, Mass.: Academic Press, 2001).

# Bibliography

Aranya, H. S. *Yoga Philosophy of Patanjali.* Albany, N.Y.: State University of New York Press, 1983.

Benson, H. *Your Maximum Mind.* New York: Random House, 1987.

Benson, H., and J. Beary. "The Relaxation Response." *Psychiatry* 37 (1974): 37–46.

Bohm, David. *Wholeness and the Implicate Order.* London: Routledge and Kegan Paul, 1980.

Borysenko, J. *Minding the Body, Mending the Mind.* Reading, Mass.: Addison-Wesley Publishing Company, 1987.

Charlton, H. *Hell-Bent for Heaven: The Autobiography of Hilda Charlton.* Lake Hill, N.Y.: Golden Quest, 1990.

Dalai Lama. *The Four Noble Truths.* London: Thorsons, 1997.

Davis, R. E. *A Guide to Kriya Yoga Practice: Discipleship Guidelines and Meditation Routines for Initiates.* Lakemont, Ga.: CSA Press, 2000.

Everly, G. S., and H. Benson. "Disorders of Arousal and the Relaxation Response: Speculation on the Nature and Treatment of Stress-Related Diseases." *International Journal of Psychosomatics* 36 (1989): 15–21.

Ganesh Anand Giri, S. S. M. "The Cycle of Synthesis." Unpublished oral teachings.

Grof, S., and C. Grof, eds. *Spiritual Emergency.* Los Angeles: Jeremy P. Tarcher, 1989.

Gupta, R .K. *A Yoga of Indian Classical Dance: The Yogini's Mirror.* Rochester, Vt.: Inner Traditions International, 2000.

Hariharananda, S. *Kriya Yoga.* Orissa, India: Swami Hariharananda Giri, 1981.

Kabat-Zinn, J. *Full Catastrophe Living.* New York: Delacorte, 1991.

Kant, I. *Critique of Reason.* London: Everyman, 1934.

Krishna, G. *Kundalini: The Evolutionary Energy in Man.* Berkeley, Calif.: Shambhala, 1971.

Lazar, S., et al. "Functional Brain Mapping of the Relaxation Response and Meditation." *NeuroReport* 11 (2000): 1581–85.

Lowenstein, K. "Meditation and Self-Regulatory Techniques." In *Handbook of Complementary and Alternative Therapies in Mental Health,* edited by Scott Shannon. Cambridge, Mass.: Academic Press, 2001.

Mascaró, Juan, trans. *The Bhagavad Gita.* New York: Penguin Books, 1962.

Neuhaus, E. B. *The Crazy Wisdom of Ganesh Baba: Psychedelic Sadhana, Kriya Yoga, Kundalini, and the Cosmic Energy in Man.* Rochester, Vt.: Inner Traditions, 2010.

Newberg, A. B., and J. Iversen. "The Neural Basis of the Complex Mental Task of Meditation: Neurotransmitter and Neurochemical Considerations." *Medical Hypotheses* 61, no. 2 (2003): 282–91.

Nityananda, S. *Kriya-Yoga: The Science of Life-Force.* New Delhi, India: Munshiram Manoharlal Publishers, 2013.

O'Brian, E. G. *The Jewel of Abundance: Finding Prosperity through the Ancient Wisdom of Yoga.* Novato, Calif.: New World Library, 2018.

Prajanananada, P. *The Yoga Sutras of Patanjali.* Vienna, Austria: Prajna Publication, 2011.

Porges, S. W. "Vagal Tone: A Physiologic Marker of Stress Vulnerability." *Pediatrics* 90, no 3 (1992): 498–504.

Porges, S. W., et al. "Infant Regulation of the 'Vagal Brake' Predicts Child Behavior Problems." *Developmental Psychobiology* 29, no. 8 (1996): 697–712.

Rahula, W. *What the Buddha Taught.* New York: Grove Press, 1959.

Rama, S., R. Ballentine, and A. Hymes. *Science of the Breath.* Honsdale, Pa.: Himalayan Institute, 1979.

Sivanada, S. *The Science of Pranayama.* Himalayas, India: The Divine Life Society, 1978.

———. *Science of Yoga.* Vol. 8 of *Raja Yoga.* Durban: Sivananda Press, 1974.

Sutherland, W. *Teachings in the Science of Osteopathy.* Portland, Ore.: Rudra Press, 1990.

Vivekananda, S. *Raja Yoga.* New York: Ramakrishna-Vivekananda Center, 1973.

Williams, P., and R. Warwick, eds. *Grey's Anatomy*, 36th ed. Philadelphia: W. B. Saunders, 1980.

Wyder, H. *Kriya Yoga: Four Spiritual Masters and a Beginner.* Steyning, U.K.: Kriya Source Publishing, 2014.

Yogananda, P. *Autobiography of a Yogi,* 6th ed. Los Angeles: Self-Realization Fellowship, 1955.

Yukteswar, S. *The Holy Science.* Los Angeles: Self-Realization Fellowship, 1977.

Zimmer, H. *Philosophies of India.* Princeton, N.J.: Princeton University Press, 1951.

# Index

Page numbers in *italics* indicate illustrations.

# About the Author

Keith G. Lowenstein, M.D., is a physician in Portland, Oregon. He works with children, adolescents, and adults with a focus on both mental and physical stress-related illness. He is board certified in psychiatry, obesity medicine, and integrative medicine. With more than thirty years of clinical experience Dr. Lowenstein has a lifelong commitment to a comprehensive approach to human health and development.

Prior to his medical training, Dr. Lowenstein began his study of the mind-body interface in 1971 with his training in Transcendental Meditation. Dr. Lowenstein's study, practice, and teaching of Kriya Yoga began in 1980 with Sri Mahant Swami Ganeshanand Saraswati Giri, a monk from the line of Paramahansa Yogananda, author of *Autobiography of a Yogi*. Dr. Lowenstein subsequently spent the next five years studying and teaching Kriya Yoga alongside Swami Ganeshanand, known as Ganesh Baba.

In order to broaden his approach to healing, Dr. Lowenstein has consistently sought out additional training in various modalities. He studied at the Mind-Body Institute with Herbert Benson, M.D., author of *The Relaxation Response* and physician at Harvard Medical School. Dr. Lowenstein was one of the first students to study with Andrew Weil, M.D., at the University of Arizona Medical School. A founding diplomate of the American Board of Integrative and Holistic Medicine (ABIHM), Dr. Lowenstein served as faculty for the early board review course. Dr. Lowenstein is also a graduate of the Helms Medical Institute in medical acupuncture.

Dr. Lowenstein has additional training in cranial osteopathy, nutrition, and naturopathy, and he utilizes mindfulness and somatic psychotherapies as well as psychodynamic and cognitive behavioral approaches in his work. He incorporates auricular acupuncture regularly into his practice with a specific emphasis on PTSD.

Dr. Lowenstein frequently presents at national and international medical conferences and is a consultant for corporations, agencies, schools, and health plans that seek to evaluate and implement individual and corporate wellness/stress-reduction programs. Due to his unique perspective and training, Dr. Lowenstein often facilitates presentations on integrative holistic health care, nutrition, stress-related illness, and Kriya Yoga.

Currently, Dr. Lowenstein maintains an integrative mental health private practice in Portland, Oregon, where he teaches Kriya Yoga and self-regulatory techniques to all ages.